More Calculated Cooking

Also by Jeanne Jones:

THE CALCULATING COOK
DIET FOR A HAPPY HEART
THE FABULOUS FIBER COOKBOOK
FITNESS FIRST: A 14-DAY DIET AND EXERCISE PROGRAM
JEANNE JONES' PARTY PLANNER AND ENTERTAINING DIARY
SECRETS OF SALT-FREE COOKING

More Calculated Cooking

By Jeanne Jones

ILLUSTRATIONS BY HOLLY ZAPP
PREFACE BY LEO P. KRALL, M.D.

101 Productions
San Francisco

In Grateful Acknowledgment
to My Publishers,
Jacqueline and Roy Killeen

Copyright © 1981 Jeanne Jones
Drawings Copyright © 1981 Holly Zapp

Printed and bound in the United States of America.
Distributed to the book trade in the United States
by Charles Scribner's Sons, New York.

Published by 101 Productions
834 Mission Street
San Francisco, California 94103

Library of Congress Cataloging in Publication Data

Jones, Jeanne.
    More calculated cooking.

    Continues The calculating cook.
    Bibliography: p.
    Includes index.
    1. Diabetes--Diet therapy--Recipes.   2. Low-
calorie diet--Recipes.   I. Title.
RC662.J68   641.5'614   80-25179
ISBN 0-89286-184-3

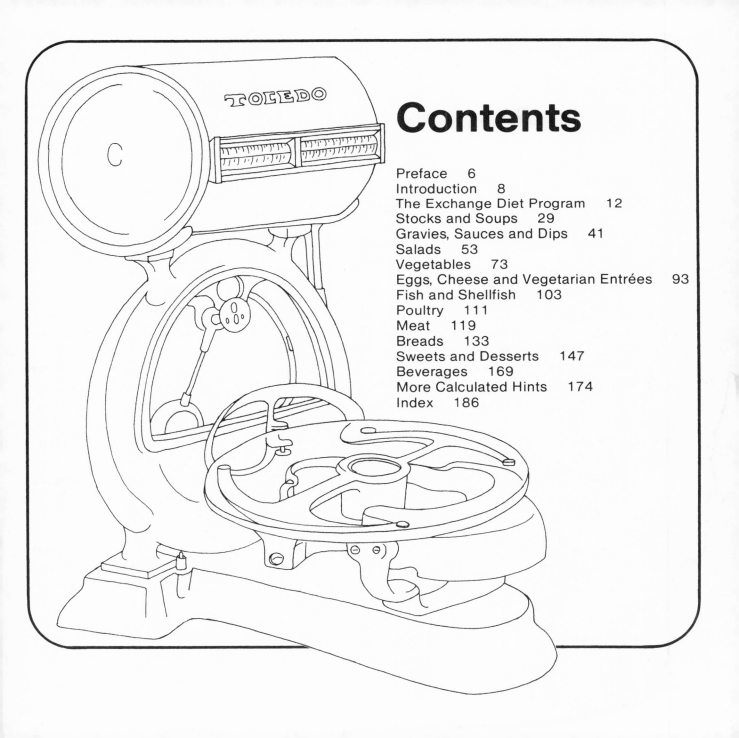

Contents

Preface

Why should anyone write a preface to someone else's book? There are lots of reasons. It may be that you owe the author a favor. You may happen to like and admire the author. The author may be very successful and you may want to share in that success. There is the rare chance that the book may really be good and useful as an exciting educational tool. On very rare occasions such as this one, all of the above may be true.

Jeanne Jones is a unique phenomenon. The world is full of diets, most of which are either followed fitfully or cheerfully ignored because of their dullness. Jeanne swims almost alone against the prevailing tide of diet methods and shows that good eating habits need not be limited to two graham crackers and a half glass of skim milk for "health's" sake. She has found ways of creating adventure in the kitchen with simple foods. At the other end of the gastronomic scale, she has made Escoffier-caliber chefs turn fresh green-bean green with envy at her scrumptious but relatively low-calorie creations.

When the former editor-in-chief of the American Diabetes Association publication *Diabetes Forecast* was struggling in an attempt to make diabetic diets more exciting, like a knight clad in an armor of cooking utensils, with a saucepan for a shield and a ladle for a sword, Jeanne Jones came to the rescue with a series of brilliant dissertations that made it possible to eat hamburgers in a crystal-chandeliered palace as well as to revel in gourmet delights at a beach picnic.

In addition to being a tirelessly energetic and wildly imaginative calculating cook, she is a frenetic world traveler. She has lived in Mexico and has munched freshwater chestnuts on the streets of Benares, India. She has discussed high-fiber diets with experts in England and carbohydrates with representatives of the developing nations in Dubrovnik, Yugoslavia. In all of these travels she has picked up suggestions, ideas and hints that have been translated into hundreds of lectures and thousands of best-selling books. Moreover, she has another charming attribute. She tests all of these recipes, perfects them and uses them.

It is not possible for all her readers to eat with Jeanne Jones at one of her dinners. The book method, however, is even better. You can invite Jeanne into your own kitchen and dining room. Living long is important, but the quality of life is just as important. Now you too can eat, drink and . . . be happy!

LEO P. KRALL, M.D.
Director, Education Division, Joslin Diabetes Foundation
Lecturer in Medicine, Harvard Medical School
Editor-in-Chief, *Diabetes Forecast* Magazine,
   American Diabetes Association, 1974-79
Associate Editor, *Metabolism*
Vice President, International Diabetes Federation, London

Introduction

Since *The Calculating Cook* was published ten years ago, I have written six other cookbooks, including a party planner and entertaining diary, and a diet and exercise book. In each of my books I have dealt with other diet modifications such as low cholesterol, low saturated fat, low sodium, higher fiber and calorie control for weight reduction. All of these modifications are simply refinements of the diabetic exchange diet. The exchange diet is nothing more than a perfectly balanced diet for all nutritional needs at the calorie level prescribed by your doctor. I like to call the exchange diet program a perfect diet because it is, in fact, the best diet in the world for everyone.

I still love to cook and to entertain just as much as I did when I wrote my first book. Over the past ten years, however, my own work schedule has become steadily more demanding. Writing books, consulting and frequent speaking engagements throughout the world have made it necessary for me to find many shortcuts in order to entertain when I am at home.

I feel even more strongly now that using your imagination in the kitchen is what makes both cooking and entertaining fun and exciting. The most important thing I want to convey in this book is how to start using your own imagination. In developing new recipes and variations of old ones I always start by thinking of variations on every other recipe I have. For example, if a soup is really good hot, I refrigerate what is left and try serving it cold. If it is just as good cold, I try jelling it and turning it into a molded salad. If the salad turns out to be a winner, I add enough meat exchanges to use it for a main course. You can see there is no limit to the number of variations possible for a recipe when you add other ingredients or leave some out. Also, as often as possible, think of food in terms of "escaping from the ordinary"—leave the mundane for other people. Just because you have never heard of serving a salad for breakfast does not mean that fruit and cottage cheese cannot be an excellent breakfast alternative, and a godsend to people who do not like the classic bacon-and-eggs approach. Nothing in the Bible tells us that eating bacon and eggs for breakfast is necessary to get to heaven; however, many cardiovascular doctors believe that bacon and eggs can indeed get you to heaven faster than fruit and low-fat cottage cheese!

So the sky is the limit—let your imagination run wild. To help you get started, I have given at least one variation for every recipe in this book. Many of these variations will show you that leftovers are indeed fabulous ingredients, and this new way of thinking about food preparation will save you money as well as time. Calories and exchanges for variations remain the same as for the main recipe unless otherwise stated.

To create your own variations by making substitutions of other ingredients, use the exchange lists in this book. Never feel that just because you don't have some of the ingredients in a recipe you can't use it. If the recipe calls for a low-fat meat exchange, go through the exchange list for a suitable substitute. Chances are you can find something else in the same exchange category that will be just as good *and* maybe even better.

When I was handed my first exchange list it was a very small piece of paper with these words at the top: "DO NOT EAT ANYTHING NOT ON THIS LIST." It was a bleak prospect to think of living the rest of my life restricted to this short, rather dull, group of foods. I have now expanded the diabetic exchange lists to include almost every known food, so there is no longer any need for anyone on this diet program to feel deprived. You will quickly see that there isn't anything you actually can't eat—it is simply a question of how much of it and when. In fact, diabetics in good control are often in better shape than their non-diabetic friends who overeat both in quantity and junk and don't get an adequate amount of exercise.

Never feel that when you are having company you have to serve something other than what is on your own diet program. Remember—it is the best diet in the world for everyone. You will find your guests will enjoy coming to your home for dinner even more when they know that they are not going to be served enormous portions of overly rich foods. Today almost everyone is health-conscious and appreciates an imaginative and delicious meal that is not loaded with unnecessary calories.

Never be discouraged if something doesn't turn out well. My philosophy is "Never apologize for a mistake in the kitchen—just rename it." No one else knows exactly what the recipe was supposed to look like or taste like in the first place. So unless it is a total disaster, chances are a new name for the dish and a positive attitude on the part of the cook will turn it into a success. Once when I was reheating broccoli for a dinner party I burned it slightly. Rather than throw it out, I called it "browned broccoli!" Another time, I made a cold soufflé that didn't jell properly, so I spooned it into custard cups and called it a mousse.

The word "calculating" means far more than simply calculating the exchanges and working with figures so that your menus are perfectly balanced each day. Being a "calculating cook" means calculating in every possible way—figuring out new and unusual ways of combining foods that are good for you, delicious, beautiful and fun to prepare. First read my book. Start using my recipes—and then get busy dreaming up new recipes of your own and becoming a *Calculating Cook* yourself.

The Exchange Diet Program

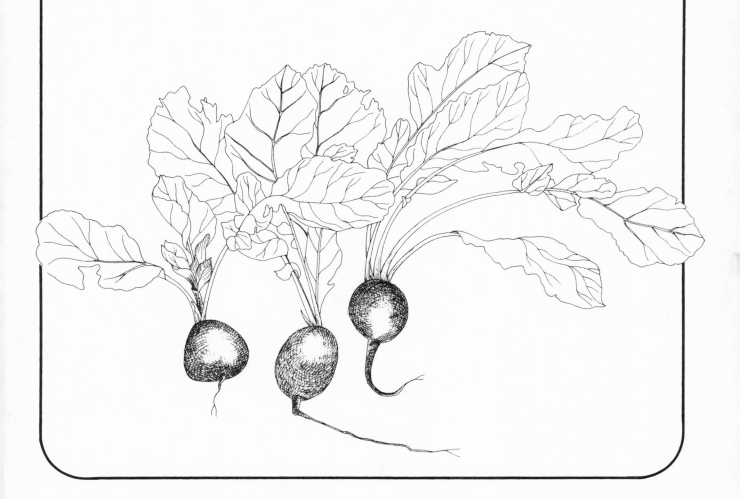

The Exchange Diet Program

The Exchange Diet Program is a system of grouping foods according to the amounts of carbohydrates, protein, fat and calories they contain. There are six basic types of foods:

1. Foods containing only carbohydrates are called FRUIT EXCHANGES or FRUIT PORTIONS.
2. Foods containing carbohydrates and small amounts of protein are called VEGETABLE EXCHANGES or VEGETABLE PORTIONS.
3. Foods containing larger amounts of carbohydrates and protein are called BREAD EXCHANGES or STARCH PORTIONS.
4. Foods containing nearly equal amounts of carbohydrates and proteins are called MILK EXCHANGES or MILK PORTIONS. They are divided into three groups: non-fat, low-fat and whole, depending upon the amount of fat each contains.
5. Foods containing protein and some fat are called MEAT EXCHANGES or PROTEIN PORTIONS. They are also divided into three groups: low-fat, medium-fat and high-fat, depending on the amount of fat each contains.
6. Foods containing mostly fat are called FAT EXCHANGES or FAT PORTIONS.

"Exchange" is the term given to a specified amount of a certain type of food. One Exchange may be "exchanged" for any other specified amount within the same group because it has the same food value and the same number of calories. For example: 1 small orange is listed as 1 Fruit Exchange; 2 apricots are also 1 Fruit Exchange. If you are allowed only 1 Fruit Exchange for lunch you may want 1 small orange or you may want only 1/2 orange and 1 apricot, which also equals 1 Fruit Exchange. It doesn't matter which fruit or fruits you choose so long as the amount you eat adds up to 1 Fruit Exchange.

The same thing is true of all the Exchange lists. The Bread Exchange list gives 1 slice of bread as 1 Bread Exchange. 1 Bread Exchange can also be 1/2 cup rice. If you are allowed only 1 Bread Exchange for lunch, you may want 1 slice of bread toasted or you may want 1/2 cup rice instead. If you want both the toast and rice, you can only have 1/2 slice toast and 1/4 cup rice, which added together equal 1 Bread Exchange.

As a general rule, trades should not be made between the different Exchange groups.

However, it is good to know which food groups can be exchanged for other food groups in cases of emergencies.

The easiest interchange between the Exchange lists is for Fruit and Bread Exchanges. Also it is the most frequently necessary for emergencies.

1 Fruit Exchange = 2/3 Bread Exchange
1 Bread Exchange = 1-1/2 Fruit Exchanges

For example: If fruit were not available, you could eat 2/3 slice of bread instead of the fruit. Or if you needed another Bread Exchange, you could eat 3 dates instead of 1/2 English muffin or 1-1/2 Fruit Exchanges instead of 1 Bread Exchange!

You can also interchange Bread Exchanges with Vegetable Exchanges.

1 Vegetable Exchange = 1/3 Bread Exchange
1 Bread Exchange = 3 Vegetable Exchanges

For example: You can substitute 1 soda cracker for 1 cup cooked broccoli or have 3/4 cup cooked peas instead of 1 slice bread.

One 8-ounce glass of low-fat milk equals 1 Low-fat Milk Exchange and may be substituted for 1 Bread Exchange plus 1 Low-fat Meat Exchange.

Or, if you don't have the milk, you may have 1 generous Fruit Exchange plus 1 Low-fat Meat Exchange. See why you often hear milk called the complete food!

Remember these interchanges are for emergencies only and should not be used all of the time.

Sound complicated? Well, it certainly did to me, but you will be amazed how quickly and easily it will become very simple and almost second nature to remember exact portions.

The following table summarizes the calorie and nutritional content of each of the Exchange categories, including percentages of carbohydrate, protein and fat calories. Because the Exchange Diet rounds numbers to the nearest whole digit to make it easier for laypersons to compute their calorie intake, the percentages shown do not always total 100 percent of the total calories in an Exchange group. If you need to keep your weight down, take particular note of the fact that a gram of fat is equal to 9 calories, while a gram of either carbohydrate or protein is equal to 4 calories. It becomes easy to see why fat will indeed make you fat faster! Drinking

alcoholic beverages is discouraged because alcohol contains 7 calories per gram and contributes nothing nutritionally; therefore you are wasting precious calories needed for nutritionally beneficial foods.

This diet allows you to measure foods rather than weighing them. Therefore, it is just as easy to eat the proper amounts when you are away from home. You will be amazed at how quickly you can sight-guess the amounts of food allowed very accurately. This allows you to eat in restaurants with very few problems.

When eating in restaurants it is always best to order "straightforward" foods. By straightforward I mean foods without any breading and either broiled, baked, steamed or poached, without added fats such as butter or oil. Always ask for your sauces and salad dressings served on the side. This way you are able to control the amount of sauce or salad dressing rather than relying upon someone else to do it for you. Usually that someone else is a bit heavy-handed. It is difficult to calculate exact exchanges even when you add your own sauces and salad dressings, not knowing exactly what is in them.

When you are a guest in someone's home, you can usually eat most of what you are served. When you have a heavily sauced entrée, simply scrape off the sauce as discreetly as possible, or if you know your host or hostess well enough, ask in advance to have your portion served without sauce. And at dessert time, for Heaven's sake don't go into your medical history! Remember what I told you in *The Calculating Cook:* Just tell your hostess that her dinner was so delicious you have already eaten too much and couldn't possibly eat one more thing! However, in banquet situations I have found that it is a good idea to always accept dessert. Push it around with your fork and leave it on your plate. If you refuse it, five other waiters will try to give you some.

Calculating Calories

When creating recipes of your own or figuring the exchange information and calories in other recipes, you will frequently have to work in fractions of exchanges. I find it is much easier to use a chart giving the exact number of calories available in fractions of exchanges rather than trying to remember all of the numbers or stopping to re-calculate each time the information is needed.

This is an exact copy of the chart I keep in my own kitchen. I suggest you copy it and put it up in your kitchen.

Menu Planning

At first we all have trouble planning menus so that all the exact amounts of everything we are supposed to be eating come out right (that is called an understatement!).

ONE EXCHANGE	CALORIES	CARBOHYDRATE		PROTEIN		FAT	
		Grams	×4 Calories	Grams	×4 Calories	Grams	×9 Calories
Fruit	40	10	40 (100%)				
Vegetable	25	5	20 (80%)	2	8 (32%)		
Bread	70	15	60 (86%)	2	8 (12%)		
Low-fat Meat	55			7	28 (51%)	3	27 (49%)
Medium-fat Meat	75			7	28 (37%)	5	45 (60%)
High-fat Meat	95			7	28 (29%)	7	63 (66%)
Fat	45					5	45 (100%)
Non-fat Milk	80	12	48 (60%)	8	32 (40%)	Tr.	
Low-fat Milk	125	12	48 (38%)	8	32 (27%)	5	45 (36%)
Whole Milk	170	12	48 (28%)	8	32 (19%)	10	90 (53%)

*See following lists for portion sizes of the exchanges.

EXCHANGE	CALORIES			
	Whole	Three-Fourths	One-Half	One-Fourth
Fruit	40	30	20	10
Vegetable	25	19	13	7
Bread	70	53	35	18
Low-fat Meat	55	42	28	14
Medium-fat Meat	75	57	38	19
High-fat Meat	95	72	48	24
Fat	45	34	23	12
Non-fat Milk	80	60	40	20
Low-fat Milk	125	94	63	32
Whole Milk	170	128	85	43

The biggest problem is that it is impossible to get away from using fractions, parts of Exchanges, in recipes. To make this problem as simple as possible I have kept all of the fractions the same throughout the book. They are all either 1/4, 1/2 or 3/4 of the whole Exchange portion.

This same menu planning guide appears in *The Calculating Cook.* I have gone a step further here, however, and have included a calorie-calculating chart to go with it so that you can easily add up the calories for fractions of exchanges without stopping to do the arithmetic each time.

An easy way to plan your menus is to always think of each Exchange as looking like this:

 1 EXCHANGE

Then as you use each part of the Exchange think of it like this:

1 EXCHANGE 3/4 LEFT

1/2 EXCHANGE 1/2 LEFT

3/4 EXCHANGE 1/4 LEFT

For example you may have 1/4 of a Bread Exchange in your main dish. So think of it like this:

1/4 EXCHANGE 3/4 LEFT

Isn't it easier to picture 3/4 of a slice of bread or 3/4 of 1/2 cup of rice this way? Or go a step further and use another 1/2 Bread Exchange in your salad (croûtons). You had this:

1/4 EXCHANGE 3/4 LEFT

now you have:

3/4 EXCHANGE 1/4 LEFT

No need to fret over how to use 1/4 Bread Exchange in a gourmet fashion. Just eat 2 tablespoons of rice or 1/4 slice of bread and forget it.

If you learn to keep this mental picture, even going through a cafeteria line will cease to be a nightmare. You first pick up a salad with 1/4 cup pineapple

1/2 FRUIT EXCHANGE

1/2 FRUIT EXCHANGE LEFT

and 1/2 cup of low-fat cottage cheese

 2 LOW-FAT MEAT EXCHANGES

Now you don't have any more Meat Exchanges left because you only have 2 for that meal, but you still have

 1/2 FRUIT EXCHANGE

 1 BREAD EXCHANGE

 1/2 MILK EXCHANGE LEFT

Then you see 1/4 cup blueberries. Great, now your Fruit Exchange looks like this:

Just like it should!

Take 1/2 pint of milk, pour 1/2 of it over your blueberries

Take 2 graham crackers

eat them with your blueberries and milk for dessert. You've had a perfectly balanced lunch.

Start using the menu programs beginning on page 176 as a guide. Look at all of them for ideas, not just the ones for your calorie level. Before long you will have fun planning your own menus easily and with imagination.

Fruit Exchange List

Each portion below equals 1 Fruit Exchange and contains approximately:

   10 grams of carbohydrate
   40 calories

  * good source of Vitamin C
 ** good source of Vitamin A
*** good source of Vitamins A and C
†† figures not available

gm. fiber	mg. chol.	mg. sodium	
1.0	0	1	Apple: 1 2 inches in diameter
.1	0	.7	Apple juice: 1/3 cup
.6	0	2	Applesauce, unsweetened: 1/2 cup
.6	0	1	Apricots, fresh: 2 medium**
.5	0	3	Apricots, dried: 3 halves**
			Avocado: see Fat Exchange List
.3	0	.5	Banana: 1/2 small
2.0	0	1	Blackberries: 1/2 cup
1.1	0	1	Blueberries: 1/2 cup
.3	0	10	Cantaloupe: 1/4 6 inches in diameter***
.3	0	1	Cherries, sweet: 10 large
††	0	2	Cranberries, unsweetened: 1 cup
.3	0	††	Crenshaw melon: 2-inch wedge
.5	0	2	Dates: 2
.5	0	2	Date "sugar": 1 tablespoon
.6	0	1	Figs, fresh: 1 large
.8	0	7	Figs, dried: 1 large
0	0	0	Fructose: 1 tablespoon
.2	0	1	Grapefruit: 1/2 4 inches in diameter*
Tr.	0	1	Grapefruit juice: 1/2 cup*
.4	0	2	Grapes: 12 large
.2	0	2	Grapes, Thompson Seedless: 20 grapes
Tr.	0	1	Grape juice: 1/4 cup
4.4	0	2	Guava: 2/3*
0	0	1	Honey: 2 teaspoons
.7	0	27	Honeydew melon: 1/4 5 inches in diameter
.4	0	††	Kiwi: 1 medium
3.0	0	6	Kumquats: 2
Tr.	0	1	Lemon juice: 1/2 cup
Tr.	0	1	Lime juice: 1/2 cup
.5	0	††	Loquats: 3
.2	0	3	Litchi nuts, fresh: 3
.9	0	3	Mango: 1/2 small**
††	0	18	Molasses, blackstrap: 1 tablespoon
.3	0	8	Nectarine: 1 medium
.5	0	1	Orange: 1 small*
.1	0	1	Orange juice: 1/2 cup*
1.0	0	3	Papaya: 1/3 medium*
1.5	0	16	Passionfruit: 1
.1	0	††	Passionfruit juice: 1/3 cup
.6	0	1	Peach: 1 medium
1.0	0	3	Pear: 1 small
.8	0	3	Persimmon: 1/2 medium
.3	0	1	Pineapple, fresh or canned without sugar: 1/2 cup
Tr.	0	1	Pineapple juice: 1/3 cup
.2	0	6	Plantain: 1/2 small
.3	0	2	Plums: 2 medium
.2	0	3	Pomegranate: 1 small
.3	0	2	Prunes, fresh or dried: 2
Tr.	0	5	Prune juice: 1/4 cup
.2	0	6	Raisins: 2 tablespoons
3.0	0	1	Raspberries: 1/2 cup
1.5	0	1	Strawberries: 3/4 cup
0	0	0	Sucrose: 1 tablespoon
.5	0	2	Tangerines: 1 large or 2 small
.5	0	1.5	Watermelon: 3/4 cup

Vegetable Exchange List

Each portion below equals 1 Vegetable Exchange, is equal to 1 cup unless otherwise specified, and contains approximately:

   5 grams of carbohydrate
   2 grams of protein
   25 calories

  *Good source of Vitamin C
 **good source of Vitamin A
***good source of Vitamins A and C
 †calories negligible when eaten raw
††figures not available

gm. fiber	mg. chol.	mg. sodium	VEGETABLES
.6	0	††	Alfalfa sprouts†
4.8	0	40	Artichoke, whole, base and ends of leaves (1 small)
1.0	0	1	Asparagus†
.7	0	4	Bean sprouts†
.8	0	40	Beets (½ cup)
1.3	0	37	Beet greens
††	0	8	Breadfruit (¼ cup)
1.5	0	22	Broccoli***†
1.6	0	16	Brussels sprouts*
.8	0	16	Cabbage*†
1.0	0	24	Carrots (medium), 1**
1.0	0	12	Cauliflower†
.6	0	100	Celery†
.7	0	100	Celery root (½ cup)
.9	0	166	Chard†
.8	0	12	Chayote
.9	0	††	Chicory**†
2.0	0	42	Chilies†
1.2	0	16	Chives***†
.9	0	56	Collard*†
1.4	0	††	Coriander (Cilantro)†
.6	0	8	Cucumber†
1.6	0	80	Dandelion greens†
1.8	8	2	Eggplant
1.2	0	10	Endive†
1.0	0	10	Escarole**†
††	0	10	Garlic (¼ cup)
.5	0	3	Green beans: see String beans
1.0	0	8	Green onion tops†
.3	0	31	Horseradish, prepared (1 tablespoon)
.5	0	††	Jerusalem artichokes (½ cup)
††	0	††	Jicama
1.2	0	48	Kale*†
.7	0	12	Leeks (½ cup)
.6	0	7	Lettuce†
1.8	0	.5	Lima beans, baby (¼ cup)
††	0	††	Mint†
.8	0	10	Mushrooms†
.9	0	12	Mustard, fresh*†
1.0	0	4	Okra
.6	0	9	Onions (½ cup)
1.2	0	††	Palm heart
1.5	0	32	Parsley***†
.75	0	.4	Peas (¼ cup)
††	0	Tr.	Pea pods, Chinese (½ cup)
1.5	0	20	Peppers, green and red*†
††	0	8	Pimiento (½ cup)
.9	0	††	Poke†
1.3	0	2	Pumpkin (½ cup)*
.7	0	20	Radishes†
.9	0	2	Rhubarb†
.7	0	4	Romaine lettuce†
1.1	0	4	Rutabagas (½ cup)
††	0	9	Shallots (½ cup)
.9	0	37	Spinach†
1.2	0	1	Squash, acorn (½ cup)
.2	0	1	Squash, Hubbard (1/2 cup)
††	0	2	Squash, spaghetti
1.2	0	6	String beans
1.2	0	2	Summer squash†
.9	0	6	Tomatoes (1 medium)
††	0	15	Tomatoes, canned in juice, unsalted (½ cup)
.1	0	282	Tomato catsup, regular (1 ½ tablespoons)
††	0	6	Tomato catsup, dietetic, low-sodium (1 ½ tablespoons)
.4	0	244	Tomato juice (½ cup)
††	0	26	Tomato juice, unsalted (½ cup)
.3	0	186	Tomato paste (2 tablespoons)
††	0	12	Tomato paste, unsalted (3 tablespoons)
.6	0	831	Tomato sauce (½ cup)
††	0	42	Tomato sauce, unsalted (½ cup)
.8	0	27	Turnips (½ cup)
.3	0	550	V-8 juice (⅔ cup)**
††	0	49	V-8 juice, unsalted (⅔ cup)**
.2	0	8	Water chestnuts (medium) (4)
.7	0	16	Watercress**†
1.4	0	1	Zucchini squash†

Bread Exchange List

Each portion below equals 1 Bread Exchange and contains approximately:
- 15 grams of carbohydrate
- 2 grams of protein
- 70 calories

**good source of Vitamin A
††figures not available

gm. fiber	mg. chol.	mg. sodium	VEGETABLES
1.4	0	3	Beans, dried, cooked, unsalted (lima, soya, navy, pinto, kidney): ½ cup
.5	0	1.5	Beans, baked, without salt or pork: ¼ cup
.6	0	1	Corn, on-the-cob: 1 4 inches long
.6	0	1	Corn, cooked and drained: ⅓ cup
.1	0	††	Hominy: ½ cup
.7	0	14	Lentils, dried, cooked: ½ cup
2.0	0	8	Parsnips: 1 small
.5	0	13	Peas, dried, cooked (black-eyed, split): ½ cup
.7	0	7	Potatoes, sweet, yams: ¼ cup**
.5	0	2	Potatoes, white, baked or boiled: 1 2 inches in diameter
.5	0	2	Potatoes, white, mashed: ½ cup
.2	0	300	Potato chips: 15 2 inches in diameter
2.6	0	4	Pumpkin, canned: 1 cup
.2	0	6	Rice, brown, cooked, unsalted: ⅓ cup
Tr.	0	3	Rice, white, cooked, unsalted: ½ cup
††	0	4	Rice, wild, cooked, unsalted: ½ cup
.2	0	564	Tomato catsup, commercial: 3 tablespoons
††	0	12	Tomato catsup, dietetic, low sodium, 3 tablespoons

gm. fiber	mg. chol.	mg. sodium	BREADS
Tr.	0	††	Bagel: ½
Tr.	0	185	Biscuit: 1 2 inches in diameter
††	0	7	Bread, low sodium: 1 slice
.1	0	139	Bread, rye: 1 slice
.4	0	136	Bread, whole wheat: 1 slice
Tr.	0	148	Bread (white and sourdough): 1 slice
Tr.	0	200	Breadsticks: 4 7 inches long
Tr.	0	116	Bun, hamburger: ½
Tr.	0	153	Bun, hot dog: ⅔
.1	0	245	Corn bread: 1 piece 1½ inches square
.3	0	††	Cracked wheat (bulgur): 1½ tablespoons
Tr.	0	140	Croutons, plain: ½ cup
††	0	7	Croutons, plain, low-sodium bread: ½ cup
Tr.	0	133	English muffin: ½
Tr.	0	1	Matzo cracker, plain: 1 6 inches in diameter
Tr.	0	222	Melba toast: 6 slices
Tr.	0	117	Muffin, unsweetened: 1 2 inches in diameter
Tr.	0	412	Pancakes: 2 3 inches in diameter
††	0	7	Pancakes, low sodium: 2 3 inches in diameter
Tr.	0	88	Popover: 1
Tr.	0	143	Roll: 1 2 inches in diameter
Tr.	0	70	Rusks: 2
.1	0	712	Spoon bread: ½ cup
.3	0	Tr.	Tortilla, corn, flour: 1 7 inches in diameter
Tr.	0	203	Waffle: 1 4 inches in diameter

gm. fiber	mg. chol.	mg. sodium	
			CEREALS
2.4	0	287	All-Bran: ½ cup
2.0	0	94	Bran Flakes: ½ cup
3.3	0	††	Bran, unprocessed rice: ⅓ cup
3.2	0	††	Bran, unprocessed wheat: ⅓ cup
.2	0	240	Cheerios: 1 cup
.2	0	††	Concentrate: ¼ cup
.1	0	178	Corn Flakes: ⅔ cup
.1	0	1	Cornmeal, cooked: ½ cup
Tr.	0	1	Cream-of-Wheat, cooked: ½ cup
.4	0	147	Grapenuts: ¼ cup
.3	0	113	Grapenut Flakes: ½ cup
.1	0	1	Grits, cooked: ½ cup
Tr.	0	165	Kix: ¾ cup
.3	0	132	Life: ½ cup
Tr.	0	1	Malt-O-Meal, cooked: ½ cup
Tr.	0	2	Maypo, cooked: ½ cup
Tr.	0	1	Matzo meal, cooked: ½ cup
.2	0	1	Oatmeal, cooked: ½ cup
.3	0	.5	Oatmeal, uncooked: ¼ cup
.2	0	92	Pep: ½ cup
.2	0	1	Puffed rice: 1½ cup
.3	0	1	Puffed wheat: 1½ cups
Tr.	0	174	Rice Krispies: ⅔ cup
.4	0	1	Shredded wheat, biscuit: 1 large
.3	0	168	Special K: 1¼ cups
.2	0	1	Steel cut oats, cooked: ½ cup
.4	0	163	Wheat Chex: ½ cup
Tr.	0	1	Wheat germ, defatted: 1 ounce or 3 tablespoons
.2	0	210	Wheaties: ⅔ cup
			FLOURS
Tr.	0	2	Arrowroot: 2 tablespoons
Tr.	0	1	All purpose: 2½ tablespoons
Tr.	0	138	Bisquick: 1½ tablespoons
3.2	0	††	Bran, unprocessed wheat: 5 tablespoons
.3	0	1	Buckwheat: 3 tablespoons
Tr.	0	1	Cake: 2½ tablespoons
.1	0	Tr.	Cornmeal: 3 tablespoons
Tr.	0	Tr.	Cornstarch: 2 tablespoons
Tr.	0	1	Matzo meal: 3 tablespoons
Tr.	0	12	Potato flour: 2½ tablespoons
.5	0	1	Rye, dark: 4 tablespoons
.6	0	1	Whole wheat: 3 tablespoons
Tr.	0	1	Noodles, macaroni, spaghetti, cooked: ½ cup
Tr.	9.4	2	Noodles, dry, egg: 3½ ounces
Tr.	3.1	1.5	Noodles, cooked, egg: 3½ ounces
			CRACKERS
Tr.	0	††	Animal: 8
Tr.	0	33	Arrowroot: 3
Tr.	0	††	Cheese tidbits: ½ cup
.2	0	88	Graham: 2
††	0	10	Low sodium: 4
Tr.	0	220	Oyster: 20 or ½ cup
Tr.	0	90	Pretzels: 10 very thin, or 1 large
Tr.	0	250	Saltines: 5, salted
Tr.	0	69	Soda: 3, unsalted
Tr.	0	192	Ritz: 6
.3	0	225	RyKrisp: 3
.3	0	130	Rye thins: 10
Tr.	0	336	Triangle thins: 14
††	0	150	Triscuits: 5
Tr.	0	††	Vegetable thins: 12
Tr.	0	276	Wheat thins: 12
			MISCELLANEOUS
1.8	0	10	Cocoa, dry, unsweetened: 2½ tablespoons
††	0	120	Fritos: ¾ ounce or ½ cup
0	26.3	40	Ice cream, low saturated fat: ½ cup
.3	0	1	Popcorn, popped, unbuttered and unsalted: 1½ cups

Low-fat Meat Exchange List

Each portion below equals 1 Low-fat Meat Exchange and contains approximately:

    7 grams of protein
    3 grams of fat
    55 calories

†† figures not available

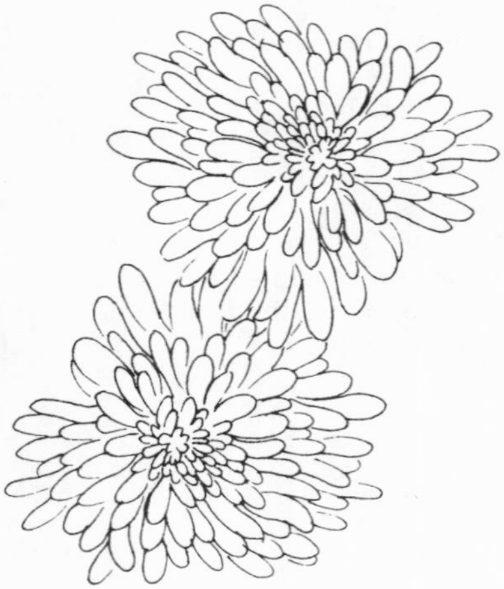

gm. fiber	mg. chol.	mg. sodium	
			CHEESE
0	2.6	234	Cottage cheese, low-fat: ¼ cup
0	1.3	90	Cottage cheese, dry curd: 1 ounce
0	††	222	Farmers': ¼ cup, crumbled, salted
0	3.0	75	Farmers': ¼ cup, crumbled, unsalted
0	3.0	††	Hoop (Bakers'): ¼ cup
0	3.0	12	Pot: ¼ cup
0	18.2	46	Ricotta, part skim: ¼ cup or 2 ounces
			EGG SUBSTITUTES
0	0	130	Liquid egg substitute: ¼ cup (sodium content varies with brands)
0	0	††	Dry egg substitute: 3 tablespoons
			CHICKEN
0	25.8	22	Broiled or roasted: 1 ounce or 1 slice 3×2×⅛ inch
0	22.4	19	Breast, without skin: ½ small, 1 ounce or ¼ cup, chopped
0	25.8	25	Leg: ½ medium or 1 ounce
			TURKEY
0	22.4	23	Meat, white, without skin: 1 ounce or 1 slice 3×2×⅛ inch
0	††	28	Meat, dark, without skin: 1 ounce or 1 slice 3×2×⅛ inch
			OTHER POULTRY AND GAME
0	30.0	25	Buffalo: 1 ounce or 1 slice 3×2×⅛ inch
0	††	22	Cornish game hen, without skin: ¼ bird or 1 ounce
0	††	20	Pheasant: 1½ ounces
0	25.8	18	Rabbit: 1 ounce or 1 slice 3×2×⅛ inch
0	††	12	Quail, without skin: ¼ bird or 1 ounce
0	††	22	Squab, without skin: ¼ bird or 1 ounce
0	††	25	Venison, lean, roast or steak: 1 ounce or 1 slice 3×2×⅛ inch

gm. fiber	mg. chol.	mg. sodium	FISH AND SHELLFISH
0	24.4	††	Abalone: 1⅓ ounces
0	18.3	112	Albacore, canned in oil: 1 ounce
0	21.4	††	Anchovy fillets: 9
0	††	1540	Anchovy paste: 1 tablespoon
0	27.1	15	Bass: 1½ ounces
0	85.7	624	Caviar: 1 ounce
0	††	††	Clam juice: 1½ cups
0	18.0	51	Clams, fresh: 3 large or 1½ ounces
0	27.0	††	Clams, canned: 1-1/2 ounces
0	18.1	31	Cod: 1 ounce
0	43.0	77	Crab, canned: 1/2 ounce
0	42.5	90	Crab, cracked, fresh: 1-1/2 ounces
0	30.2	110	Flounder: 1-2/3 ounces
0	55.0	††	Frog legs: 2 large or 3 ounces
0	18.1	30	Halibut: 1 ounce or 1 piece 2×2×1 inch
0	27.0	††	Herring, pickled: 1¼ ounces
0	††	2207	Herring, smoked: 1¼ ounces
0	31.0	90	Lobster, fresh: 1½ ounces, ¼ cup or ¼ small lobster
0	36.0	90	Lobster, canned, unsalted: 1½ ounces
0	23.0	31	Oysters, fresh: 3 medium or 1½ ounces
0	25.5	171	Oysters, canned: 1½ ounces
0	27.1	39	Perch: 1½ ounces
0	27.1	38	Red snapper: 1½ ounces
0	18.4	14	Salmon: 1 ounce
0	16.0	235	Salmon, canned: 1½ ounces
0	18	††	Salmon, smoked (lox): 1½ ounces
0	24.4	33	Sand dabs: 1½ ounces
0	40.0	108	Sardines: 4 small
0	††	26	Sardines, unsalted: 4 small
0	23.0	112	Scallops: 3 medium or 1½ ounces
0	48.0	60	Shrimp, fresh: 5 medium
0	64.0	††	Shrimp, canned: 5 medium or 1½ ounces

gm. fiber	mg. chol.	mg. sodium	
0	30.0	44	Sole: 1⅔ ounces
0	27.1	††	Swordfish: 1½ ounces
0	27.1	11	Trout: 1½ ounces
0	18.1	10	Tuna, fresh: 1 ounce
0	††	370	Tuna, canned in oil: ¼ cup
0	††	25	Tuna, unsalted, water packed (dietetic): ¼ cup
0	27.1	32	Turbot: 1½ ounces
			BEEF
0	41.8	26	Flank steak: 1½ ounces
0	31.3	17	Rib roast: 1 ounce, ¼ cup, chopped, or 1 slice 3×2×⅛ inch
0	30.0	17	Steak, very lean (filet mignon, New York, sirloin, T-bone): 1 ounce or 1 slice 3×2×⅛ inch
0	††	21	Tripe: 1 ounce or 1 piece 5×2 inches
			LAMB
0	28.0	20	Chops, lean: ½ small chop or 1 ounce
0	27.7	20	Roast, lean: 1 ounce, 1 slice 3×2×⅛ inch, or ¼ cup, chopped
			PORK
0	25.3	264	Ham: 1 ounce or 1 slice 3×2×⅛ inch
			VEAL
0	28.7	23	Chop: ½ small or 1 ounce
0	29.0	23	Cutlet: 1 ounce or 1 slice 3×2×⅛ inch
0	28.7	23	Roast: 1 ounce or 1 slice 3×2×⅛ inch

Medium-fat Meat Exchange List

Each portion below equals 1 Medium-fat Meat Exchange and
contains approximately:

7 grams of protein
5 grams of fat
75 calories   †† figures not available

gm. fiber	mg. chol.	mg. sodium	
			CHEESE
0	8.4	130	Cottage cheese, creamed: ¼ cup
0	16.0	††	Feta: 1 ounce
0	17.4	227	Mozzarella: 1 ounce
0	14.8	163	Parmesan: ¼ cup, ⅔ ounce or 4 tablespoons
0	29.1	46	Ricotta, regular: ¼ cup or 2 ounces
0	14.8	247	Romano: ¼ cup, ⅔ ounce or 4 tablespoons
			EGGS
0	250.0	59	Eggs, medium: 1
0	0	47	Egg white: 1 (not a whole portion)
0	250.0	12	Egg yolk: 1 (not a whole portion)
			CHICKEN
0	††	16	Gizzard: 1 ounce
0	††	20	Heart: 1 ounce
0	211.4	17	Liver: 1 ounce

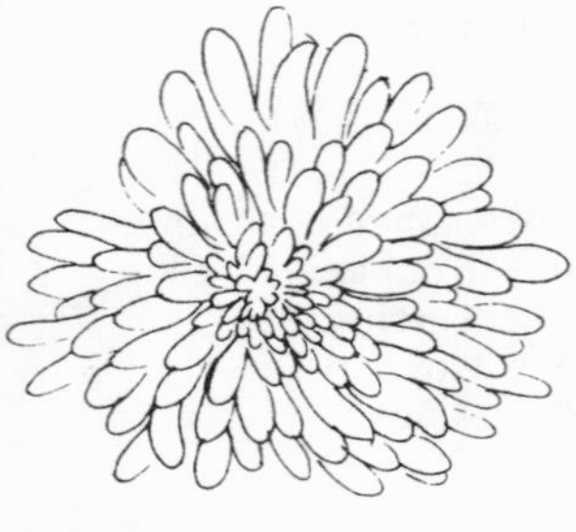

gm. fiber	mg. chol.	mg. sodium	
			BEEF
0	571.4	54	Brains: 1 ounce
0	26.0	298	Corned beef, canned: 1 ounce or 1 slice 3×2×⅛ inch
0	30.3	14	Hamburger, very lean (4 ounces raw = 3 ounces cooked): 1 ounce
0	42.8	30	Heart: 1 ounce or 1 slice 3×2×⅛ inch
0	107.1	72	Kidney: 1 ounce or 1 slice 3×2×⅛ inch
0	124.1	59	Liver: 1 ounce or 1 slice 3×2×⅛ inch
0	††	17	Tongue: 1 slice 3×2×⅛ inch
			PORK
0	25.3	343	Canadian bacon: 1 slice 2½ inches in diameter, ¼ inch thick
0	25.0	18	Chops, lean: ½ small chop or 1 ounce
0	††	19	Heart: 1 ounce
0	124.1	30	Liver: 1 ounce
0	25.0	18	Roast, lean: 1 ounce, 1 slice 3×2×⅛ inch or ¼ cup, chopped
			VEAL
0	124.1	30	Calves' liver: 1 ounce or 1 slice 3×2×⅛ inch
0	71.4	33	Sweetbreads: 1 ounce, ¼ pair or ¼ cup, chopped
0	28.7	22	Roast, lean: 1 ounce, ¼ cup, chopped, or 1 slice 3×2×⅛ inch
			VEGETABLES
0	0	2	Tofu (soybean curd): 4 ounces, ½ cup or 1 slice 2×2×1-½ inches

High-fat Meat Exchange List

Each portion below equals 1 High-fat Meat Exchange and contains approximately:
- 7 grams of protein
- 7 grams of fat
- 95 calories

††figures not available

gm. fiber	mg. chol.	mg. sodium	
			CHEESE
0	28.4	193	American: 1 ounce
0	21.16	510	Blue: 1 ounce or ¼ cup, crumbled
0	30.1	193	Cheddar: 1 ounce
0	††	10	Cheddar, low sodium: 1 ounce (sodium content varies with brands)
0	29.1	204	Edam: 1 ounce
0	21.0	271	Liederkranz: 1 ounce
0	18.0	204	Monterey Jack: 1 ounce
0	25.0	204	Muenster: 1 ounce
Tr.	18.2	465	Pimiento cheese spread: 1 ounce
0	24.0	465	Roquefort: 1 ounce or ¼ cup, crumbled
0	21.0	††	Stilton: 1 ounce or ¼ cup, crumbled
0	28.0	85	Swiss: 1 ounce
			COLD CUTS
0	25.9	266	Bologna: 1 ounce or 1 slice 4½ inches in diameter, ⅛ inch thick
0	††	264	Liverwurst: 1 slice 3 inches in diameter, ¼ inch thick
0	25.9	340	Spam: 1 ounce
0	25.9	425	Salami: 1 ounce or 1 slice 4-½ inches in diameter, ⅛ inch thick
0	25.9	228	Vienna sausage: 2½ sausages or 1 ounce

gm. fiber	mg. chol.	mg. sodium	
			DUCK
0	††	21	Roasted, without skin: 1 ounce or 1 slice 3×2×⅛ inch
0	††	28	Wild duck, without skin: 1 ounce
			BEEF
0	31.3	17	Brisket: 1 ounce
0	25.9	508	Frankfurters: 1 (8 to 9 per pound)
0	31.3	18	Short ribs, very lean: 1 rib or 1 ounce
			PEANUT BUTTER
.3	0	156	Peanut butter, regular: 2 tablespoons
.3	0	6	Peanut butter, unsalted: 2 tablespoons
			PORK
			Bacon: see Fat Exchange List
0	25.9	250	Sausage, 2 small or 1 ounce
0	25.3	19	Spareribs, without fat: meat from 3 medium or 1 ounce

Fat Exchange List

Each portion below equals 1 Fat Exchange and contains approximately:
    5 grams of fat
    45 calories

†† figures not available

gm. fiber	mg. chol.	mg. sodium	
.8	0	1	Avocado: ⅛ 4 inches in diameter
0	7.0	209	Bacon, crisp: 1 slice
0	12.0	39	Butter: 1 teaspoon
0	††	.3	Butter, unsalted: 1 teaspoon
1.2	††	5	Caraway seeds: 2 tablespoons
1.2	††	5	Cardamom seeds: 2 tablespoons
0	0	4	Chocolate, bitter: ⅓ ounce or ⅓ square
0	10.0	35	Cream cheese: 1 tablespoon
0	20.0	5	Cream, heavy, whipping: 1 tablespoon
0	20.0	12	Cream, light, coffee: 2 tablespoons
0	17.0	18	Cream, half-and-half: 3 tablespoons
0	16.0	12	Cream, sour: 2 tablespoons
0	0	32	Cream, sour, imitation: 2 tablespoons (Imo, Matey)
0	0	35	Margarine, polyunsaturated: 1 teaspoon
0	0	.8	Margarine, polyunsaturated, unsalted: 1 teaspoon
0	2.6	25	Mayonnaise: 1 teaspoon
0	0	0	Oils, polyunsaturated: 1 teaspoon
.6	††	125	Olives, ripe: 5 small
††	††	384	Olives, green: 4 medium
.8	††	3	Poppy seeds: 1½ tablespoons
.2	††	††	Pumpkin seeds: 1½ teaspoons

gm. fiber	mg. chol.	mg. sodium	
			Salad dressings, commercial:
Tr.	††	59	Blue cheese: 1 teaspoon
Tr.	††	95	Blue cheese, diet, sugar 1 teaspoon
Tr.	††	57	Caesar: 1 teaspoon
Tr.	††	77	French: 1 teaspoon
Tr.	††	74	Italian: 1 teaspoon
Tr.	††	64	Italian, diet: 1 teaspoon
Tr.	††	48	Roquefort: 1 teaspoon
Tr.	††	44	Thousand Island, diet: 1 teaspoon
Tr.	††	33	Thousand Island, egg-free: 1 teaspoon
			Sauces, commercial:
Tr.	††	††	Bearnaise: 1 teaspoon
Tr.	††	28	Hollandaise: 1 teaspoon
Tr.	††	61	Tartar: 1 teaspoon
.2	0	4	Sesame seeds: 2 teaspoons
.2	0	3	Sunflower seeds: 1½ teaspoons
			NUTS, UNSALTED
.3	0	.5	Almonds: 7
.2	0	.5	Brazil nuts: 2
.2	0	2	Cashews: 7
.5	0	5	Coconut, fresh: 1 piece 1×1×⅜ inch
.3	0	5	Coconut, shredded, unsweetened: 2 tablespoons
1.2	0	.5	Filberts: 5
1.2	0	.5	Hazelnuts: 5
.1	0	††	Hickory nuts: 7 small
.3	0	††	Macadamia nuts: 2
.4	0	1	Peanuts, Spanish: 20
.4	0	1	Peanuts, Virginia: 10
.3	0	Tr.	Pecans: 6 halves
.2	0	††	Pine nuts: 1 tablespoon
.1	0	††	Pistachio nuts: 15
.2	0	††	Soy nuts, toasted: 3 tablespoons
.2	0	.5	Walnuts, black: 5 halves
.2	0	.5	Walnuts, California: 5 halves

Non-fat Milk Exchange List

Each portion below equals 1 Non-fat Milk Exchange and contains approximately:

12 grams of carbohydrate
8 grams of protain
   trace of fat
80 calories   †† figures not available

gm. fiber	mg. chol.	mg. sodium	
0	7.8	280	Buttermilk: 1 cup
0	††	155	Milk, powdered, skim, dry: 3 tablespoons
0	1.7	115	Milk, powdered, skim, mixed: ¼ cup
0	2.3	127	Milk, skim, non-fat: 1 cup
0	††	121	Milk, skim, instant: 1 cup
0	2.3	165	Milk, evaporated, skim: ½ cup
0	††	75	Sherbet: 1 cup
0	††	116	Yogurt, plain, non-fat: 1 cup

Low-fat Milk Exchange List

Each portion below equals 1 Low-fat Milk Exchange and contains approximately:

12 grams of carbohydrate
 8 grams of protein
 5 grams of fat
125 calories

gm. fiber	mg. chol.	mg. sodium	
0	15.5	150	Milk, low-fat, 2% fat: 1 cup
0	17.0	115	Yogurt, plain, low-fat: 1 cup

Whole Milk Exchange List

Each portion below equals 1 Whole Milk Exchange and contains approximately:

12 grams of carbohydrate
 8 grams of protein
10 grams of fat
170 calories   †† figures not available

gm. fiber	mg. chol.	mg. sodium	
0	26.0	136	Ice milk: 1 cup
0	32.7	120	Milk, whole: 1 cup
0	32.7	149	Milk, evaporated, whole: ½ cup
0	††	6	Milk, low-sodium Lonolac liquid: 1 cup
0	††	114	Yogurt, plain, whole: 1 cup

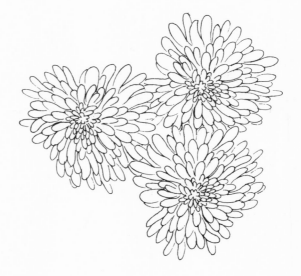

Herbs, Spices, Seasonings, Etc.

Calories are negligible and need not be counted in the following list; however, many of these foods are extremely high in sodium and must be calculated very carefully.

†† figures not available

gm. fiber	mg. chol.	mg. sodium	
0	0	250	Baking powder: 1 teaspoon
0	0	Tr.	Baking powder, low sodium: 1 teaspoon
0	0	1360	Baking soda: 1 teaspoon
††	0	10	Bakon Yeast: 1 teaspoon (12 calories)
0	0	Tr.	Bitters, Angostura: 1 teaspoon
0	0	425	Bouillon cube, beef (fat free): 1½-inch cube or 4 grams
0	0	10	Bouillon cube, beef (fat free and salt free): 1½-inch cube or 4 grams
0	0	5	Bouillon cube, chicken (fat free and salt free): 1½-inch cube or 4 grams
Tr.	0	306	Capers: 1 tablespoon
††	0	294	Chutney: 1 tablespoon (Crosse & Blackwell's, Major Grey's)
0	0	1	Coffee: 1 cup
0	0	Tr.	Extracts: 1 teaspoon
0	0	4	Gelatin, unsweetened: 1 envelope (1 scant tablespoon)
0	0	0	Liquid smoke: 1 teaspoon
Tr.	0	63	Mustard, prepared: 1 teaspoon (French's)
Tr.	0	811	Pickles: 1 2 ounce, without sugar
0	0	6	Rennet tablets: 1 ounce
0	0	2200	Salt: 1 teaspoon
0	0	2077	Soy sauce: 1 ounce (2 tablespoons)
0	0	6	Tabasco sauce: ¼ teaspoon
0	0	Tr.	Vinegar, cider: 1 tablespoon
0	0	5	Vinegar, red wine: 1 tablespoon
0	0	5	Vinegar, white wine: 1 tablespoon
0	0	58	Worcestershire sauce: 1 tablespoon (Lea & Perrins)

gm. fiber	mg. chol.	mg. sodium	
.4	0	2	Allspice, ground: 1 teaspoon
.4	0	1	Allspice, whole: 1 teaspoon
††	0	Tr.	Aniseed: 1 teaspoon
.2	0	Tr.	Basil: 1 teaspoon
††	0	Tr.	Bay leaf: 1 leaf
.2	0	4	Celery seed, ground: 1 teaspoon
.2	0	2	Celery seed, whole: 1 teaspoon
††	0	31	Chili powder, seasoned: 1 teaspoon
.3	0	Tr.	Cinnamon, ground: 1 teaspoon
††	0	3	Cloves, ground: 1 teaspoon
††	0	1	Cloves, whole: 1 teaspoon
.4	0	Tr.	Coriander, ground: 1 teaspoon
.1	0	Tr.	Cumin seed: 1 teaspoon
††	0	1	Curry powder: 1 teaspoon
.4	0	Tr.	Dill seed: 1 teaspoon
††	0	Tr.	Dill weed: 1 teaspoon
.4	0	1	Fennel seed: 1 teaspoon
Tr.	0	1	Garlic powder: 1 teaspoon
††	0	1	Ginger, ground: 1 teaspoon
††	0	Tr.	Juniper berries: 1 teaspoon
††	0	Tr.	Lemon peel, dried: 1 teaspoon
††	0	Tr.	Lemon peel, fresh: 1 teaspoon
Tr.	0	2	Mace, ground: 1 teaspoon
Tr.	0	Tr.	Marjoram, dried: 1 teaspoon
Tr.	0	Tr.	Mint, dried: 1 teaspoon
††	0	Tr.	Mustard seed: 1 teaspoon
Tr.	0	Tr.	Nutmeg, ground: 1 teaspoon
.1	0	2	Onion powder: 1 teaspoon
††	0	Tr.	Oregano, dried: 1 teaspoon
.4	0	1	Paprika, ground: 1 teaspoon
.1	0	5	Parsley flakes: 1 teaspoon
.2	0	Tr.	Pepper, black: 1 teaspoon
††	0	Tr.	Pepper, cayenne: 1 teaspoon
††	0	698	Pepper, lemon: 1 teaspoon (Durkee's)
.1	0	Tr.	Pepper, white: 1 teaspoon
.2	0	Tr.	Rosemary, dried: 1 teaspoon
††	0	Tr.	Saffron, powdered: 1 teaspoon
.1	0	Tr.	Sage, dried: 1 teaspoon
.2	0	Tr.	Savory, dried: 1 teaspoon
.1	0	Tr.	Tarragon, dried: 1 teaspoon
.1	0	Tr.	Thyme, dried: 1 teaspoon
.1	0	1	Turmeric, ground: 1 teaspoon

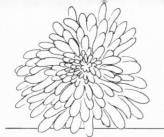

Alcoholic Beverages

Whether you are allowed alcoholic beverages in your diet should be decided between you and your doctor. There is no question that weight loss/maintenance is simplified greatly by not drinking, as liquor of all types is high in calories. Also, as you will notice by the figures given, many alcoholic beverages are also high in sodium.

A good way to think of a cocktail, highball or glass of wine is to visualize the drink as a slice of bread with a pat of butter on it. This image may help one to refrain from having another drink more than anything else does.

There is another problem with drinking on a restricted diet. Alcohol can lead to waiting too long before eating, eating too much or eating something forbidden on the diet. Most doctors, however, consider cooking with wines completely acceptable. Wine adds very little food value to each portion, and all the alcohol is cooked away before the food is eaten.

C= calories
GC= grams of carbohydrates

gm. fiber	mg. chol.	mg. sodium	
0	0	17	Ale, mild, 8 oz. = 98 C, 8 GC
0	0	8	Beer, 8 oz. = 114 C, 11 GC

WINES

gm. fiber	mg. chol.	mg. sodium	
0	0	3	Champagne, brut, 3 oz. = 75 C, 1 GC
0	0	3	Champagne, extra dry, 3 oz. = 87 C, 4 GC
0	0	4	Dubonnet, 3 oz. = 96 C, 7 GC
0	0	4	Dry Marsala, 3 oz. = 162 C, 18 GC
0	0	4	Sweet Marsala, 3 oz. = 152 C, 23 GC
0	0	4	Muscatel, 4 oz. = 158 C, 14 GC
0	0	4	Port, 4 oz. = 158 C, 14 GC
0	0	4	Red wine, dry, 3 oz. = 69 C, under 1 GC
0	0	4	Sake, 3 oz. = 75 C, 6 GC
0	0	4	Sherry, domestic, 3½ oz. = 84 C, 5 GC
0	0	4	Dry vermouth, 3½ oz. = 105 C, 1 GC
0	0	4	Sweet vermouth, 3½ oz. = 167 C, 12 GC
0	0	4	White wine, dry, 3 oz. = 74 C, under 1 GC

LIQUEURS AND CORDIALS

gm. fiber	mg. chol.	mg. sodium	
0	0	2	Amaretto, 1 oz. = 112 C, 13 GC
0	0	2	Crème de Cacao, 1 oz. = 101 C, 12 GC
0	0	2	Crème de Menthe, 1 oz. = 112 C, 13 GC
0	0	2	Curacao, 1 oz. = 100 C, 9 GC
0	0	2	Drambuie, 1 oz. = 110 C, 11 GC
0	0	2	Tia Maria, 1 oz. = 113 C, 9 GC

SPIRITS

Bourbon, brandy, Cognac, Canadian whiskey, gin, rye, rum, scotch, tequila and vodka are all carbohydrate free! The calories they contain depend upon the proof.

gm. fiber	mg. chol.	mg. sodium	
0	0	Tr.	80 proof, 1 oz. = 67 C
0	0	Tr.	84 proof, 1 oz. = 70 C
0	0	Tr.	90 proof, 1 oz. = 75 C
0	0	Tr.	94 proof, 1 oz. = 78 C
0	0	Tr.	97 proof, 1 oz. = 81 C
0	0	Tr.	100 proof, 1 oz. = 83 C

Stocks & Soups

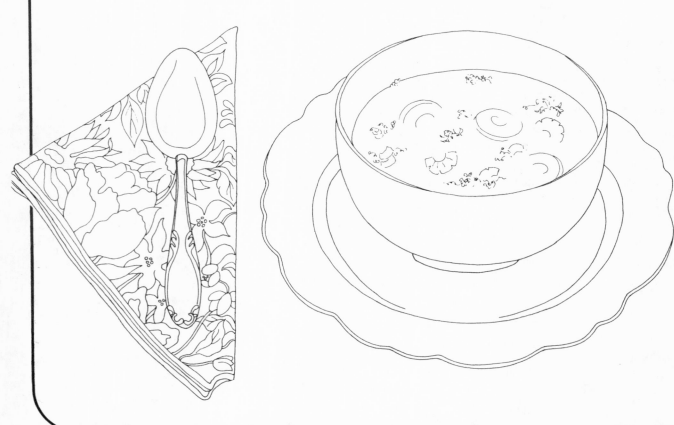

Stocks and Consommés

Making your own stocks takes so little time and makes such a difference in the flavors of your sauces and gravies that I feel it is an extremely important facet of food preparation even in a quick and easy approach to cooking.

I always put all of my poultry carcasses and scraps in one bag and beef bones and scraps in another and freeze them. (Lean ham and pork bones do not make good all-purpose stocks because their flavor is too strong.) Then, when I have the time, I put them in a stock pot. If you do not have the facilities for making your own stock or room for storing it, keep canned stock in the refrigerator. This way each time you open a new can of stock you can more easily remove all of the fat than you can if it is kept at room temperature. I feel that canned stocks are closer to homemade than bouillon cubes. In emergencies, however, dissolve bouillon cubes or powdered stock base in boiling water and proceed with the recipe.

Beef Stock

3 pounds beef or veal bones
1 pound beef, cut of choice (optional)
2 carrots, scraped and cut into pieces
2 celery stalks, without leaves
1 onion, cut in half
1 tomato, cut in half
3 garlic cloves
2 parsley sprigs
2 whole cloves
1/4 teaspoon crushed dried thyme
1/4 teaspoon crushed dried marjoram
1 bay leaf
10 peppercorns
1 teaspoon salt
Defatted beef drippings, page 41 (optional)

1. Put the bones and enough cold water to cover by 1 inch in a large soup kettle. Bring to a boil.
2. Simmer slowly for 5 minutes, then remove and discard any scum that has formed on the surface.
3. Add the meat, vegetables and spices and enough additional cold water to cover by 1 inch.
4. Cover, leaving the lid ajar about 1 inch to allow the steam to escape. Simmer very slowly for at least 5 hours (10 hours is even better).
5. When the stock is finished cooking, strain it and allow it to come to room temperature. Refrigerate, uncovered, overnight. The next morning remove and discard the fat that has hardened on the surface.
6. After removing every bit of fat, warm the stock until it becomes liquid. Strain the liquid and add salt to taste. If the flavor is too weak, boil to evaporate more of the water and concentrate the strength.
7. Store the stock in the freezer, putting some of it in ice cube trays for individual servings (2 cubes = 1/4 cup). The stock may also be stored in a tightly covered container for not more than 2 days in the refrigerator.

Makes about 2-1/2 quarts (10 cups)
Free food
Calories negligible

VARIATION:

CHICKEN STOCK: Substitute 3 pounds of chicken parts (wings, backs, etc.), for the beef or veal bones and 1 whole stewing chicken (optional) for the pound of meat. Omit the tomato, thyme and marjoram and the defatted beef drippings. Proceed as directed in the recipe.

Chicken Giblet Stock

Hearts, gizzards, livers and
  necks from 2 or 3 chickens
1 celery stalk, cut into pieces
1 carrot, scraped and cut into
  pieces
1 onion, cut into quarters
2 bay leaves
1/4 teaspoon crushed dried
  basil
1 teaspoon salt
4 peppercorns

1. Put all of the ingredients in
a large saucepan with enough
cold water to cover by 1 inch.
Bring to a boil.
2. Simmer slowly for 5 minutes, then remove and discard
any scum that has formed on
the surface.
3. Cover, leaving the lid ajar
about 1 inch to allow steam to
escape. Simmer very slowly
for 3 hours.
4. When the stock is finished
cooking, strain it, discarding
the vegetables. Remove the
giblets, chop, cover and refrigerate, reserving them for another use or for adding to the
stock later. Allow the stock to
come to room temperature,
then refrigerate it, uncovered,
overnight. The next morning,
remove and discard the fat
that has hardened on the
surface.
5. After removing every bit of
fat, warm the stock until it
becomes liquid. Strain the liquid
and add salt to taste. If the
flavor is too weak, boil to
evaporate more of the water
and concentrate the strength.
6. Return the chopped giblets
to the pot, if desired, and heat
through.
  Note: This stock is delicious
served over steamed rice. Add
the giblets to the stock and
make it a complete meal (1
cup chopped giblets = 4 low-
fat meat exchanges).

Makes 1-1/2 to 2 quarts (6 to 8 cups)
Free food
Calories negligible

VARIATION:

TURKEY GIBLET STOCK: Substitute the heart, gizzard, liver
and neck from 1 turkey for the
chicken parts. Add 1 garlic
clove, 1/8 teaspoon crushed
dried thyme, 1/8 teaspoon
crushed dried marjoram and
defatted turkey drippings, page
41 (optional). Proceed as directed in the recipe.

Chicken Consommé

4 egg whites
2 quarts (8 cups) cold Chicken
  Stock, page 29
2 bay leaves
2 parsley sprigs
4 green onion tops, chopped
2 carrots, chopped
Salt to taste
2 envelopes (2 tablespoons)
  unflavored gelatin (optional)

1. Beat the egg whites with a
wire whisk until they are slightly
foamy.
2. Add 2 cups of the cold
stock to the egg whites and
beat together lightly.

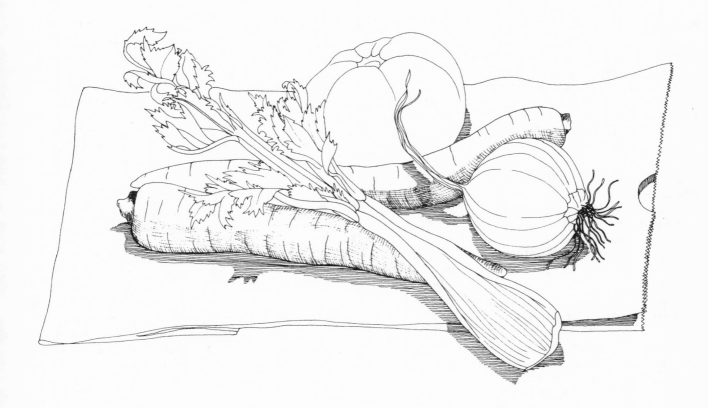

3. Put the remaining 6 cups of stock in a saucepan with all of the remaining ingredients, bring to a boil and remove from the heat.

4. Slowly pour the egg white-stock mixture into the hot stock, stirring with the wire whisk as you do.

5. Put the saucepan back on very low heat and stir gently until it starts to simmer. Put the pan half on the heat and half off so that it is barely simmering (or use a heat deflector) and turn the pan around every few minutes. Simmer for 40 minutes.

6. Let the consommé cool slightly. Line a colander or a strainer with 2 or 3 layers of damp cheesecloth and ladle the consommé through the cheesecloth. Allow it to drain undisturbed until it has all seeped through.

Makes 2 quarts (8 cups)
Free food
Calories negligible

VARIATION:

BEEF CONSOMME: Substitute 2 quarts of Beef Stock, page 29, for the Chicken Stock.

Soups

From the standpoint of using your imagination, soup is the ideal proving ground. Anything and everything can be soup. You can put vegetables in a blender or food processor and add enough stock to purée them to a soup consistency, or you can simply chop them into bite-sized pieces and heat them with enough stock, milk or juice to turn them into a soup-like presentation. Soup also can be an almost calorie-free first course or a hearty hot or cold entrée.

The presentation of soup also has almost endless variety. Cold soup can be served in chilled bowls, icers or hollowed-out fruits and vegetables such as melon halves, grapefruit halves or squash or artichoke bowls. Hot soups can be served in bowls or soup plates, or ladled from a steaming cauldron into mugs. Remember, use your imagination!

Cold Cucumber Soup

2 medium cucumbers, peeled and finely chopped
Salt
4 cups (1 quart) buttermilk
1 teaspoon fructose
1/2 teaspoon dry mustard
1/2 teaspoon ground cumin
1/2 teaspoon salt
1/4 teaspoon freshly ground black pepper
Chopped parsley for garnish (optional)

1. Place the cucumbers in a non-metal container and sprinkle lightly with salt. Cover and allow to stand for at least 1 hour. Pour off the liquid and set the cucumbers aside.

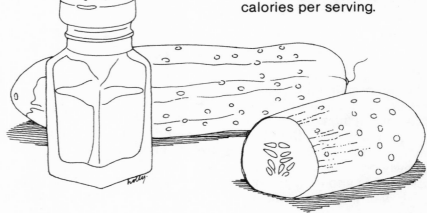

2. Combine all of the remaining ingredients, except the parsley, in a non-metal container and mix well.
3. Add the cucumbers to the other ingredients and mix well. Refrigerate, covered, until chilled.
4. Pour into 6 chilled bowls or icers and sprinkle parsley over each serving, if desired.

Makes 6 (1 cup) servings
Each serving contains approximately:
3/4 non-fat milk exchange
60 calories

VARIATION: Substitute 1 teaspoon of curry powder for the cumin and add one 8-ounce can crushed pineapple packed in natural juice, undrained, to the basic soup. Mix well. Add 1/4 fruit exchange and 10 calories per serving.

Cold Curried Grapefruit Soup

2 cups fresh grapefruit juice, unstrained
1 tablespoon quick-cooking tapioca
1/8 teaspoon salt
1/2 teaspoon date "sugar" or fructose
1/4 teaspoon curry powder
1/2 cup plain low-fat yogurt
Ground cinnamon for garnish

1. Combine all of the ingredients, except the yogurt and ground cinnamon, in a saucepan and allow to stand for 5 minutes.
2. Put the pan on medium heat and bring to a boil, stirring frequently. As soon as it boils, remove from the heat and cool to room temperature.
3. Cover and refrigerate until cold. Just before serving, stir the yogurt into the chilled soup, mixing thoroughly.
4. Pour into 4 chilled bowls or icers and sprinkle the top of each serving with ground cinnamon.

Makes 4 servings
Each serving contains approximately:
1 fruit exchange
40 calories

VARIATION:

COLD CURRIED ORANGE SOUP: Substitute orange juice for the grapefruit juice.

Cold Smoked Salmon Soup
(An Unusual Version of Lox and Bagels)

1 envelope (1 tablespoon) unflavored gelatin
2 tablespoons cold water
1/4 cup water, boiling
2 cups chicken stock
1 cup low-fat milk
1/2 cup sour cream
1/4 cup finely chopped onion
8 ounces smoked salmon, finely chopped
Finely chopped parsley for garnish

1. Soften the gelatin in the cold water for 5 minutes. Add the boiling water and stir until the gelatin is completely dissolved.
2. Place the gelatin mixture, chicken stock, milk, sour cream, onion and half the salmon in a blender container and blend until thoroughly mixed.
3. Pour the mixture into a large bowl and add the remaining smoked salmon. Mix well, cover and chill thoroughly.
4. Pour into 8 chilled bowls or icers and sprinkle parsley over each serving.

I like to serve this soup in icers with thinly sliced and toasted bagels on the side. I love lox and bagels for brunch, served with sour cream, thinly sliced onions and parsley. Now I have discovered this way to serve lox and bagels as a starter course for luncheons and dinner parties. It is an unusual presentation and much lower in calories than the classic approach.

Makes 8 servings
Each serving contains approximately:
1/2 fat exchange
1 low-fat meat exchange
78 calories

VARIATION:

COLD TUNA SOUP: Substitute one 7-ounce can water-packed tuna, drained and finely chopped, for the smoked salmon.

Spinach Soup

2 cups chicken stock
One 10-ounce package frozen
  chopped spinach, thawed
1/4 cup finely chopped onion
1/2 cup sour cream
1/2 cup plain low-fat yogurt
1/4 cup finely chopped chives
  or green onion tops for
  garnish

1. Bring the chicken stock to a boil in a saucepan. Add the spinach and onion and return to a boil.
2. Remove from the heat and cool slightly.
3. Pour the mixture into a blender container and blend until puréed. Add the sour cream and yogurt and blend until smooth.
4. If you wish to serve this soup hot, reheat to desired temperature, but do not boil. If you wish to serve it cold, refrigerate, covered, and then serve in chilled bowls. Garnish each serving with chopped chives.

Makes 6 servings
Each serving contains approximately:
3/4 fat exchange
1/4 vegetable exchange
41 calories

VARIATIONS:

BROCCOLI SOUP: Substitute one 10-ounce package of frozen chopped broccoli, thawed, for the spinach.

OYSTERS ROCKEFELLER SOUP: Add one 8-ounce can of oysters, drained, in step 1. (Reserve the liquid from the can to mix with hot milk for a wonderful low-calorie oyster bisque.) Add 1 low-fat meat exchange and 55 calories per serving.

Sherried Pea Soup

2 cups fresh or frozen peas
1 cup chicken stock
1/8 teaspoon salt
Dash white pepper
1 cup non-fat milk
2 tablespoons sherry
1/2 teaspoon freshly grated
  lemon rind for garnish

1. Combine the peas, chicken stock, salt and white pepper in a saucepan. Bring to a boil, cover and cook until the peas are tender, about 5 minutes.
2. Remove from the heat and cool slightly.
3. Pour the peas and all of the liquid from the pan into a blender container. Add the milk and sherry and blend until smooth.
4. Pour the soup into a large bowl, cover and refrigerate until chilled.
5. Pour into 8 chilled bowls and sprinkle each serving with a pinch of lemon rind.
  This soup is nice served in the place of a salad, before a hot meal.

Makes 8 (1/2 cup) servings
Each serving contains approximately:
1-1/4 vegetable exchanges
32 calories

VARIATION:

HOT SHERRIED PEA SOUP: Instead of refrigerating the soup, heat to serving temperature, being careful not to boil.

Spiced Apple Soup

1 envelope (1 tablespoon)
  unflavored gelatin
3 cups unsweetened apple
  juice
1/8 teaspoon ground cloves
1/8 teaspoon ground allspice
1/4 teaspoon ground cinnamon
1/2 teaspoon vanilla extract
1/2 cup plain low-fat yogurt
6 apple slices for garnish
  (optional)
6 cinnamon sticks for garnish
  (optional)

1. Soften the gelatin in 2 tablespoons of the apple juice for 5
minutes.
2. Put the remaining apple juice
in a saucepan and add the
cloves, allspice, cinnamon and
vanilla extract.
3. Bring the apple juice mixture to a boil. Remove from
the heat and add the softened
gelatin, stirring until the gelatin is completely dissolved. Allow the apple juice mixture to
come to room temperature.

4. Transfer to a large bowl,
cover and refrigerate until
chilled and slightly thickened.
Add the yogurt and mix thoroughly.
5. Serve in 6 chilled bowls.
Garnish each serving with an
apple slice and a cinnamon
stick, if desired. (Or top each
serving with 1-1/2 teaspoons
of sour cream; add 1/4 fat exchange and 11 calories per
serving.)

Makes 6 (1/2 cup) servings
Each serving contains approximately:
1-1/2 fruit exchanges
60 calories

VARIATION:

SPICED APPLE DESSERT: Soften
2 envelopes (2 tablespoons) of
unflavored gelatin in 1/4 cup
of the apple juice for 5 minutes and proceed with the
recipe. Spoon the more firmly
jelled spiced apple mixture into
6 sherbet glasses or dessert
dishes. Garnish with apple
slices and cinnamon sticks.

Chicken-Mushroom Soup

4 cups chicken stock
2 teaspoons corn oil margarine
1 cup (4 ounces) fresh mushrooms, sliced
1/4 teaspoon crushed dried
  chervil
1 teaspoon fresh lemon juice
Minced watercress for garnish

1. Place the chicken stock in
a saucepan and bring to a boil.
2. In a skillet, melt the margarine and add the sliced
mushrooms. Sauté until just
tender. Do not overcook.
3. Add the mushrooms, chervil
and lemon juice to the chicken
stock and mix thoroughly.
4. Serve in small bowls and
garnish with watercress.

Makes 6 servings
Each serving contains approximately:
3/4 fat exchange
34 calories

VARIATION:

MATZO BALL-MUSHROOM SOUP:
Add 12 Matzo Balls, page 139,
to the soup and heat to serving
temperature. Add 1 bread exchange and 70 calories per
serving (2 matzo balls per
serving).

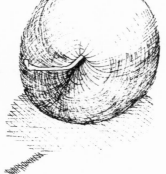

Peanut Butter Soup

4 teaspoons corn oil
  margarine
1/2 medium onion, finely
  chopped
2-1/2 tablespoons all-purpose
  flour
1 teaspoon curry powder
1/4 teaspoon salt
1 cup boiling chicken stock
1/2 cup unhomogenized
  smooth peanut butter
3 cups non-fat milk

1. Melt the margarine in a saucepan. Add the chopped onion and cook until the onion is clear and tender. *Do not brown.*
2. Add the flour, curry and salt and cook, stirring constantly, for 3 minutes.
3. Slowly add the boiling chicken stock, stirring constantly.
4. Add the peanut butter and continue to stir until slightly thickened and the peanut butter is completely melted.

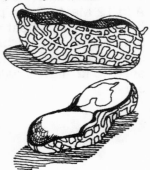

5. Slowly add the milk and heat to serving temperature. *Do not boil.* Serve hot or cool to room temperature, cover and refrigerate until thoroughly chilled.

Makes 6 servings
Each serving contains approximately:
3/4 high-fat meat exchange
3/4 fat exchange
1/2 non-fat milk exchange
146 calories

VARIATIONS:

PEANUT BUTTER-FRUIT SOUP: Any fruit is good with this soup. I particularly like chopped apples, but puréed bananas and apple-sauce are also delicious. Add the fruit to the soup just before serving either hot or cold. Check the fruit exchange list for the calories the fruit will add per serving.

PEANUT BUTTER-CHICKEN SOUP: For a wonderful luncheon entrée, add 1-1/2 cups of chopped cooked chicken or turkey to Peanut Butter-Fruit Soup and heat through. Add 1 low-fat meat exchange and 55 calories per serving.

Calcutta Consommé

3 cups chicken stock
3 cups tomato juice
1 tablespoon fresh lemon juice
1/8 teaspoon salt
1/8 teaspoon curry powder
2 whole cloves
8 thin lemon slices for garnish

1. Combine all of the ingredients, except the lemon slices, in a saucepan and bring to a boil. Reduce the heat and simmer, uncovered, for 10 minutes.
2. Pour into 8 soup bowls and place a thin lemon slice on top of each.

Makes 8 servings
Each serving contains approximately:
1 vegetable exchange
25 calories

VARIATION:

CALCUTTA SHRIMP CONSOMME: Add 3/4 pound cooked baby shrimp at the end of step 1 and simmer just until heated through. Add 1 low-fat meat exchange and 55 calories per serving.

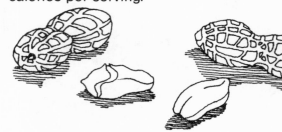

Beet Borscht

3 cups cooked beets, sliced
1 teaspoon garlic powder
1/2 teaspoon salt
1/8 teaspoon freshly ground
   black pepper
3/4 teaspoon ground allspice
1-1/2 cups buttermilk
1-1/2 cups non-fat milk
1 tablespoon freshly grated
   orange rind
2 tablespoons sour cream for
   garnish (optional)
6 lemon wedges for garnish

1. Combine all of the ingredients, except the sour cream and lemon wedges, in a blender container and blend until smooth.
2. Pour the contents of the blender container into a saucepan and heat to serving temperature. *Do not boil.*
3. Pour into 6 soup bowls and put 1 teaspoon of sour cream on top of each serving if desired. Garnish each serving with a lemon wedge.

Makes 6 servings
Each serving contains approximately:
1 vegetable exchange
1/2 non-fat milk exchange
65 calories

VARIATION:

COLD BEET BORSCHT: After blending, refrigerate until cold and serve in chilled bowls or icers. You can also reserve 1 cup of the beets, cut them in julienne and add them to the chilled soup.

Garden Soup

6 cups chicken stock
1 onion
1 whole clove
1 celery stalk, without leaves
1 bay leaf
1/4 teaspoon crushed dried
   thyme
1/2 cup watercress, chopped
1 cup fresh spinach leaves,
   chopped
1/8 teaspoon freshly ground
   black pepper
1/2 teaspoon fresh lemon juice
3 tablespoons plain low-fat
   yogurt

1. Pour the chicken stock into a large saucepan.
2. Stick the clove in the onion and add it to the chicken stock. Add the celery, bay leaf and thyme.
3. Bring to a boil, reduce the heat and simmer, covered, for 1 hour.
4. Remove the clove and bay leaf and discard.
5. Put the ingredients from the saucepan into a blender container and blend until smooth. Add the watercress, spinach, pepper and lemon juice and blend until the vegetables are chopped to the desired size.
6. Serve immediately or cool to room temperature, cover, refrigerate until thoroughly chilled and serve cold. (If reheated, the spinach and watercress lose their tangy fresh flavor.) Just before serving, hot or cold, put a small dollop of yogurt on top of each serving.

Makes 8 servings
Each serving contains approximately:
1 vegetable exchange
25 calories

VARIATION:

GARDEN CLAM CHOWDER: Add two 8-ounce cans of minced clams and all the juice from the cans to the soup after the soup is blended. Add 1 low-fat meat exchange and 55 calories per serving.

Mexican Corn Soup

1 tablespoon corn oil margarine
1/2 cup minced onion
One 16-ounce can peeled
   tomatoes, diced, juice reserved
1/4 cup all-purpose flour
1/2 teaspoon salt
1/2 teaspoon chili powder
1-1/2 teaspoons ground
   cumin
3 cups boiling chicken stock
1 cup non-fat milk, scalded
One 8-1/2-ounce can sweet
   corn, undrained

1. Melt the margarine in a
saucepan. Add the minced
onion and cook until the onion
is clear and tender, about 5
minutes.
2. Add the diced tomatoes and
can juice and mix well.
3. Combine the flour, salt, chili
powder and cumin and slowly
add it to the tomato mixture,
stirring constantly. Bring to a
simmer and cook, continuing
to stir constantly, for 3 minutes.

4. Remove from the heat and
add the boiling chicken stock,
stirring rapidly with a wire whisk
until completely blended.
5. Add the hot milk and the
corn and liquid.
6. Return to medium heat and
simmer slowly for 10 minutes,
stirring frequently to prevent
scorching.

Makes 6 servings
Each serving contains approximately:
1/2 fat exchange
1/2 vegetable exchange
1 bread exchange
106 calories

VARIATION: Add 3 cups of
chopped cooked chicken, heat
to serving temperature and
serve as the main course. Add
2 low-fat meat exchanges and
110 calories per serving.

Vegetable Soup

1 potato, peeled and diced
1 medium onion, diced
1 celery stalk, diced
1 large carrot, scraped and
   diced
1/2 cup fresh or frozen peas
5 cups water
1/4 cup finely chopped parsley
One 16-ounce can tomatoes,
   undrained
1-1/2 teaspoons salt
1/4 teaspoon freshly ground
   black pepper
1 bay leaf (optional)

1. Combine all of the ingredients in a large saucepan.
2. Bring to a boil, reduce the
heat, cover and simmer for 1
hour.
3. Remove the bay leaf and
serve.

Makes 8 servings
Each serving contains approximately:
1 vegetable exchange
25 calories

VARIATIONS:

• Use chicken or beef stock instead of water and adjust salt accordingly.

HAMBURGER SOUP: Add 4 cups (1 pound) of lean ground beef, cooked and thoroughly drained, to the soup before serving. Use beef stock in place of the water in the original recipe. Add 2 low-fat meat exchanges and 110 calories per serving.

CHICKEN SOUP: Add 4 cups (1 pound) of chopped cooked chicken to the soup before serving. Use chicken stock in place of the water in the original recipe. Add 2 low-fat meat exchanges and 110 calories per serving.

ALPHABET SOUP: Add 1 cup of alphabet macaroni to the soup during the last 15 minutes of cooking. Add 1/2 bread exchange and 35 calories per serving.

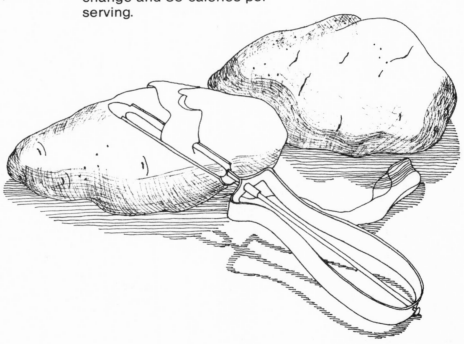

Gravies, Sauces & Dips

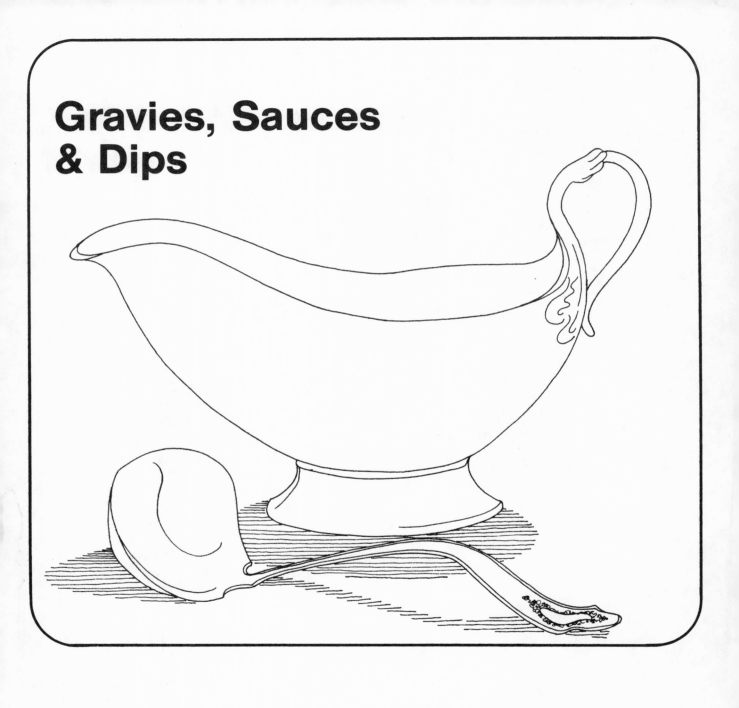

Gravies, Sauces and Dips

Sauce making can be the most time-consuming part of cooking. Also, when prepared classically, gravies, sauces and dips vie with desserts for being the foods highest in calories.

In this section of the book you will find quick and easy recipes that are also low in calories. A few of them, such as the defatted drippings and the skinny gravies, were also included in *The Calculating Cook.* They appear here because there is no way to improve upon them with respect to saving time or reducing calories.

Defatted Drippings

If you love gravy but don't eat it because it's *fat, fat, fat,* then one of your problems is solved. Just defat your drippings.

All drippings are defatted in the same manner. After cooking your roast beef, leg of lamb, chicken, turkey or whatever, remove it from the roasting pan and pour the drippings into a bowl. Put the bowl in the refrigerator until the drippings are cold and all of the fat has solidified on the top. Remove the fat and you have defatted drippings.

Now, if you are in a hurry to serve your roast beef *au jus,* just put the drippings in the freezer instead of the refrigerator. (Put the roast in the oven to keep it warm.) After about 20 minutes you can remove the fat, heat the *jus* and serve. Freeze any defatted drippings you are not using for the meal. They can be added to stocks for extra flavor and are good for making low-calorie gravies.

Skinny Beef Gravy

1 cup defatted beef drippings, preceding, or 1 cup concentrated beef stock
1 tablespoon cornstarch or arrowroot
2 tablespoons minced onion, browned, or 1 tablespoon dehydrated onion flakes (optional)

1. Heat the defatted drippings in a saucepan. As soon as they become liquid, put a little of the liquid in a cup and stir in the cornstarch to form a smooth paste.
2. Pour the cornstarch mixture into the saucepan, blending well.

3. Add the browned onion, if desired, and simmer until the gravy thickens slightly, stirring occasionally.

Note: Beef Stock, page 29, can be stored in ice-cube trays in the freezer and used for individual servings of this gravy. For one serving use 2 stock "ice cubes," 1/4 teaspoon cornstarch or arrowroot and 1 teaspoon minced onion, browned, or 1/2 teaspoon dehydrated onion flakes (optional).

Makes approximately 1 cup
Free food
Calories negligible

VARIATIONS:

SKINNY CHICKEN GRAVY: Use defatted chicken drippings in place of the beef drippings.

SKINNY TURKEY GRAVY: Use defatted turkey drippings in place of the beef drippings.

SKINNY GIBLET GRAVY: Use Chicken or Turkey Giblet Stock, page 30, in place of the beef drippings.

MUSHROOM GRAVY: Add 1/2 cup sliced mushrooms sautéed lightly in 2 teaspoons corn oil margarine in step 3. Add 1/2 fat exchange and 23 calories per each 1/4 cup of gravy.

Sauer Family Cream
(Calorie-reduced Sour Cream)

1 cup low-fat cottage cheese
2 tablespoons buttermilk
2 teaspoons fresh lemon juice

1. Put all of the ingredients in a blender container and blend until completely smooth. Even when you think it's smooth enough, blend it a little longer for a better result.

Makes 1 cup
1/4 cup contains approximately:
1 low-fat meat exchange
55 calories

VARIATIONS:

SEASONED SAUER FAMILY CREAM: Add 1 teaspoon powdered beef stock base.

ALL-PURPOSE DIP: Add 1/4 teaspoon curry powder and 2 teaspoons grated onion.

CURRY DIP: Add 1/2 teaspoon curry powder, 1/8 teaspoon ground ginger and 2 teaspoons grated onion.

MEXICAN DIP: Add 1/2 teaspoon chili powder, 1/4 teaspoon ground cumin, 1/4 teaspoon garlic powder and a dash of Tabasco sauce (optional).

ONION DIP: Add 1 teaspoon powdered beef stock base to the blender container and blend until smooth. Put in a bowl and add 2 tablespoons of dehydrated minced onions and mix well.

DESSERT DIP: Substitute 1 tablespoon non-fat milk for the buttermilk. Add 2 tablespoons fructose, 1-1/2 teaspoons vanilla extract and 1/2 teaspoon ground cinnamon (optional). Add 1/2 fruit exchange and 20 calories per 1/4 cup.

CLAM DIP: Add 2 teaspoons prepared horseradish, 1-1/2 teaspoons Worcestershire sauce, 1/2 teaspoon garlic powder and a dash of Tabasco sauce to the blender container and blend until smooth. Put in a bowl and add one 8-ounce can minced clams, drained, and mix well. Add 1-1/2 low-fat meat exchanges and 83 calories per 1/4 cup.

Jelled Milk

1 envelope (1 tablespoon) unflavored gelatin
2 tablespoons cold water
1/4 cup boiling water
1 cup non-fat milk

1. Soften the gelatin in the cold water for 5 minutes. Add the boiling water and stir until the gelatin is completely dissolved.
2. Add the milk and mix well.
3. Place the gelatin-milk mixture in a covered container in the refrigerator. When it is jelled, it is ready to use.
4. To serve, mix jelled milk with an equal amount of non-fat milk in a blender container and use over fruit or cereal. The thick, creamy consistency makes the milk seem richer.

You can mix the original ingredients with 2 cups of non-fat milk instead of only 1 cup. It is easier, however, to mix the gelatin mixture with only 1 cup and then add the second cup during the blending.

Makes 1 cup
1 cup contains approximately:
1 non-fat milk exchange
80 calories

VARIATION: Use buttermilk in place of the non-fat milk, with no change in exchanges or calories. If you use low-fat milk or whole milk, 1 cup Jelled Milk will equal 1 low-fat milk exchange and 125 calories, or 1 whole milk exchange and 170 calories.

Whipped "Cream"

2/3 cup evaporated skim milk
2 teaspoons unflavored gelatin
2 tablespoons cold water
1/4 cup boiling water

1. Pour the skim milk into a bowl and place in the freezer for about 30 minutes.
2. Soften the gelatin in the cold water in a saucepan for 5 minutes. Add the boiling water and stir until the gelatin is completely dissolved; set aside.
3. Beat the chilled skim milk until very thick. Gradually add the gelatin mixture and beat until the mixture forms soft peaks.
4. Serve immediately. (This can be refrigerated up to 1 hour but no longer without losing its whipped consistency.)

Makes 4 cups
1/2 cup contains approximately:
1/4 non-fat milk exchange
20 calories

VARIATION:

WHIPPED SWEET "CREAM": Add 2 tablespoons fructose and 1 teaspoon vanilla extract to the skim milk with the gelatin mixture. This will add 1/2 fruit exchange and 20 calories per 1/2 cup.

Basic White Sauce
(Béchamel Sauce)

2 cups non-fat milk
1 tablespoon corn oil margarine
2-1/2 tablespoons sifted all-purpose flour
1/8 teaspoon salt

1. Put the milk in a saucepan on low heat and bring to the boiling point.
2. In another saucepan, melt the margarine and add the flour, stirring constantly. Cook, stirring, for 3 minutes. *Do not brown.*
3. Remove the flour-margarine mixture from the heat and add the simmering milk all at once, stirring constantly with a wire whisk.
4. Put the sauce back on low heat and cook slowly for 15 minutes, stirring occasionally. If you wish a thicker sauce, cook it a little longer.
5. Add the salt and mix thoroughly. If there are lumps in the sauce (though there shouldn't be any by this method), whirl it in a blender container until smooth.

Makes 1-1/2 cups
3/4 cup contains approximately:
1-1/2 fat exchanges
1/2 bread exchange
1 non-fat milk exchange
183 calories

1-1/2 cups contain approximately:
3 fat exchanges
1 bread exchange
2 non-fat milk exchanges
365 calories

VARIATIONS:

MORNAY SAUCE: When the sauce has thickened, add an additional 1/2 cup non-fat milk, 1/2 cup grated Gruyère or Swiss cheese, 1/8 teaspoon ground nutmeg and 1/8 teaspoon white pepper. Heat, stirring, until the cheese is completely melted. Makes 2 cups. One cup contains approximately 1-1/2 fat exchanges, 1/2 bread exchange, 1-1/4 non-fat milk exchanges, 1 high-fat meat exchange and 298 calories.

CHEDDAR CHEESE SAUCE: When the sauce has thickened, add an additional 1/2 cup non-fat milk, 1/8 teaspoon white pepper, 1/4 teaspoon dry mustard, and 1/2 cup grated sharp cheddar cheese. Makes 2 cups sauce. One cup contains approximately 1-1/2 fat exchanges, 1/2 bread exchange, 1-1/4 non-fat milk exchanges, 1 high-fat meat exchange and 298 calories.

Mock Mayonnaise

1 cup low-fat cottage cheese
2 tablespoons corn oil
1 tablespoon red wine vinegar
1/2 teaspoon salt
1/2 teaspoon dry mustard
Dash freshly ground black
  pepper (optional)

1. Combine all of the ingredients in a blender container
and blend until smooth.
2. Cover and refrigerate for at
least 24 hours before using.

Makes 1 cup
1/4 cup contains approximately:
1-1/2 fat exchanges
1 low-fat meat exchange
123 calories

VARIATION: Substitute fresh
lemon juice for the red wine
vinegar.

Dill Sauce

1/2 cup mayonnaise
1 cup plain low-fat yogurt
1/2 teaspoon salt
1 teaspoon dried tarragon
1-1/2 tablespoons dried dill
  weed

1. Combine the mayonnaise,
yogurt and salt in a mixing
bowl and mix thoroughly with
a wire whisk.
2. Crush the tarragon and dill
weed thoroughly in a mortar
with a pestle. Add the crushed
herb mixture to the other ingredients and mix thoroughly.
  This sauce is best if prepared 2 days before you plan
to use it.

Makes 1-1/2 cups sauce
2 tablespoons contain approximately:
2 fat exchanges
90 calories

VARIATION:

TARRAGON SAUCE: Increase the
tarragon to 1 tablespoon and
omit the dill weed.

Herbed Mustard

1 cup prepared brown mustard
1 tablespoon crushed dried
  tarragon
3/4 teaspoon crushed dried
  basil
3/4 teaspoon crushed dried
  oregano
1 tablespoon red wine vinegar

1. Combine all of the ingredients and mix thoroughly.
2. Refrigerate for at least 24
hours before using.

Makes approximately 1 cup
1 tablespoonful contains approximately:
Free food
Calories negligible

VARIATION: Substitute regular
or Dijon-style mustard for the
brown mustard.

Raisin Mustard Sauce

1/4 cup raisins
1 cup water
1/2 cup non-fat milk
4 teaspoons dry mustard
1/4 cup cider vinegar
2 eggs, lightly beaten, or 1/2
  cup liquid egg substitute
1 tablespoon corn oil margarine

1. Combine the raisins and water in a saucepan. Bring slowly to a boil, reduce the heat and simmer, uncovered, for 20 minutes.
2. Combine the cooked raisins and all of the liquid in the pan with the milk in a blender container and blend until the raisins are completely puréed.
3. Pour the milk-raisin mixture back into the saucepan. Combine the dry mustard and vinegar and mix until the mustard is completely dissolved, then add to the raisin mixture in the saucepan.
4. Add the beaten eggs to the saucepan and mix thoroughly.
5. Slowly bring the sauce to a boil over low heat, stirring constantly with a whisk. When the mixture comes to a boil, remove from the heat and place the margarine on top of the mixture. Do not stir.
6. Cool the sauce to room temperature and then mix thoroughly.

  This sauce is marvelous with New England Boiled Dinner, but it is also good on many other things.

Makes 1-1/2 cups
1/4 cup contains approximately:
1/4 medium-fat meat exchange
1/4 fruit exchange
1/2 fat exchange
52 calories

VARIATION:

DATE MUSTARD SAUCE: Substitute 1/4 cup chopped pitted dates for the raisins.

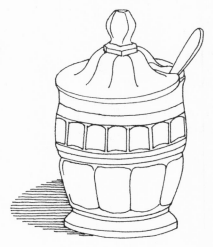

Chutney

1 pound (3 medium) tart green apples, peeled, cored and diced (2-1/2 cups)
1 medium onion, diced
1/2 cup finely chopped dried figs (5 figs)
1/4 cup raisins
1 cup cider vinegar
3/4 cup fructose
1 teaspoon salt
1/2 teaspoon ground mustard seeds
1/2 teaspoon chili powder
1-1/2 teaspoons ground ginger
1/4 teaspoon cayenne pepper
1 tablespoon pickling spices, tied in a cheesecloth bag

1. Combine all of the ingredients in a large saucepan. Bring to a boil, reduce the heat and simmer slowly, uncovered, for 2 hours.
2. Cool to room temperature. Remove and discard the cheesecloth bag containing the spices. Store, covered, in the refrigerator.

Makes 2 cups
2 tablespoons contain approximately:
1-1/2 fruit exchanges
60 calories

VARIATION:

CHUTNEY CHEESE: Combine 2 cups Chutney with 1 cup Sauer Family Cream, page 42, and mix well. Two tablespoons contain 1 fruit exchange, 1/4 low-fat meat exchange and 54 calories. Chutney Cheese is a wonderful hors d'oeuvre spread for crackers, makes a delicious sandwich spread and is an unusual dessert dip for fresh fruit.

Curried Cranberry Sauce

4 cups (1 pound) fresh cranberries
3 cups orange slices
1 cup fresh orange juice
1 cup raisins
1 teaspoon salt
1 teaspoon curry powder
1/4 teaspoon ground ginger
1/2 cup fructose

1. Combine all of the ingredients, except the fructose, in a large saucepan and bring to a boil.
2. Reduce the heat, cover and simmer for 15 to 20 minutes, or until the cranberries pop open.
3. Remove from the heat, cool to room temperature and stir in the fructose.
4. Refrigerate in a tightly covered container for at least 24 hours before serving.

This is a delightfully different cranberry sauce to serve with your traditional holiday meals.

Makes 6 cups
1/4 cup contains approximately:
1 fruit exchange
40 calories

VARIATION:

HAWAIIAN CURRIED CRANBERRY SAUCE: Substitute three 8-ounce cans of pineapple chunks packed in natural juice and all the juice from the cans, for the oranges and orange juice. Calorie and exchange differences negligible in 1/4 cup.

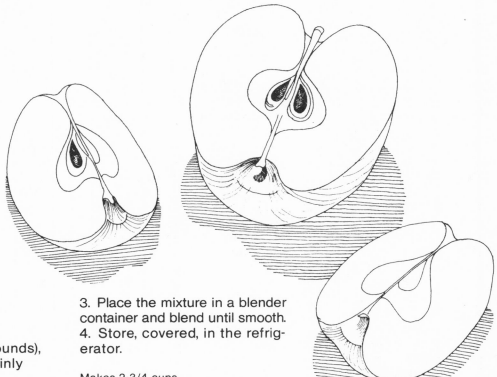

Fresh 'n Natural Apple Butter

6 medium apples (2 pounds),
  peeled, cored and thinly
  sliced (8 cups)
1 cup unsweetened apple juice
1 teaspoon ground cinnamon
1/2 teaspoon ground allspice
1/4 teaspoon ground cloves

1. Combine all of the ingredients in a large saucepan and
bring to a boil. Reduce the
heat and simmer, uncovered,
for 12 minutes, stirring occasionally.
2. Remove from the heat and
cool slightly.

3. Place the mixture in a blender
container and blend until smooth.
4. Store, covered, in the refrigerator.

Makes 2-3/4 cups
1/4 cup contains approximately:
1 fruit exchange
40 calories

VARIATION:

APPLE-RAISIN BUTTER: After the
apple butter is blended to a
smooth consistency, add 1/3
cup raisins and blend for a few
more seconds or until the raisins
are coarsely chopped. Add 1/2
fruit exchange and 20 calories
per 1/4 cup.

Apple Cider Sauce

6 medium apples (2 pounds), peeled, cored and thinly sliced (8 cups)
1 cup unsweetened apple cider
1 teaspoon ground cinnamon
1/2 teaspoon ground allspice
1/4 teaspoon ground cloves

1. Combine all of the ingredients in a large saucepan and bring to a boil. Reduce the heat and simmer, uncovered, for 12 minutes, stirring occasionally.
2. Remove from the heat and cool slightly. Place in a blender container and blend until smooth.
3. Store, covered, in the refrigerator.

This is a marvelous sauce for meat and poultry, and it is also a good dessert sauce served over fruit or cake.

Makes 2-3/4 cups
1/4 cup contains approximately:
1-1/2 fruit exchanges
60 calories

VARIATION:

CHUNKY APPLE-CIDER SAUCE: Use the same ingredients, but dice the apples into small pieces before cooking and omit the blending.

Secret Spaghetti Sauce

Two 29-ounce cans tomato sauce
4 cups (1 quart) water
1 large onion, finely chopped
2 garlic cloves, minced
1/4 teaspoon salt
1/4 teaspoon freshly ground black pepper
1 teaspoon crushed dried oregano
1 teaspoon crushed dried basil

1. Combine all of the ingredients in a large saucepan and bring to a boil.
2. Reduce the heat and simmer, uncovered, for at least 2 hours.

Makes approximately 6 cups (1-1/2 quarts)
1/2 cup contains approximately:
2 vegetable exchanges
50 calories

VARIATIONS:

SECRET SPAGHETTI MEAT SAUCE: Add 2 cups of cooked lean ground round at the end of the cooking period. Makes 8 cups. Add 1/2 low-fat meat exchange and 28 calories for each 1/2 cup serving.

SECRET SPAGHETTI CHEESE SAUCE: Add 2 cups of grated cheddar cheese at the end of the cooking period and heat just until melted. Add 1 high-fat meat exchange and 95 calories per 1/2 cup.

Christmas Dip

2 cups chopped cooked broccoli
1/2 cup tomato juice
6 tablespoons low-fat cottage cheese
1 tablespoon fresh lemon juice
1/2 teaspoon curry powder
1/2 teaspoon garlic powder
1/8 teaspoon ground ginger
One 2-ounce jar pimientos, chopped

1. Combine all of the ingredients, except the pimientos, in a blender container and blend until smooth.
2. Pour into a mixing bowl. Add the chopped pimientos and mix thoroughly.

This dip, served with raw vegetables, makes a delicious low-calorie hors d'oeuvre or appetizer.

Makes 2 cups
1/4 cup contains approximately:
1 vegetable exchange
25 calories

VARIATION:

POPEYE'S CHRISTMAS DIP: Substitute 2 cups of chopped cooked spinach for the chopped broccoli.

Bean Dip

One 16-ounce can refried
  beans
3/4 cup shredded sharp
  cheddar cheese
1/4 teaspoon salt
1/2 teaspoon onion powder
1/2 teaspoon ground cumin
1/2 teaspoon chili powder
1/2 teaspoon Tabasco sauce
Non-fat milk (optional)

1. Combine all of the ingredients and mix well.
2. If you wish a creamier consistency, thin with a little non-fat milk.

This dip is better if made several hours or the day before you plan to serve it. Serve as an hors d'oeuvre with Toasted Tortilla Chips.

Makes 3 cups
1/4 cup contains approximately:
1/2 bread exchange
1/4 high-fat meat exchange
59 calories

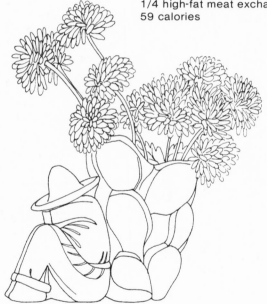

VARIATIONS:

TORTILLA SANDWICH: Spread 1/4 cup of the bean dip evenly on a soft corn tortilla. Fold the tortilla in half and wrap it in aluminum foil. Heat in a 350°F oven for 10 to 15 minutes. This is a delicious and unusual sandwich. Add 1 bread exchange and 70 calories.

MEXICAN BEAN OMELET: Use 1/4 cup of the bean dip as a filling for a 2-egg omelet. Add 2 medium-fat meat exchanges and 150 calories. Serve with warm tortillas or Toasted Tortilla Chips for a Mexican breakfast.

Spinach Spread

Two 10-ounce packages frozen
   chopped spinach, thawed
1 cup (1/2 pint) sour cream
1 tablespoon powdered beef
   stock base
1/4 cup dehydrated minced
   onion
1/2 cup finely chopped parsley
1/2 cup finely chopped green
   onions
1 teaspoon crushed dried dill
   weed
1/4 teaspoon garlic powder

1. Put the thawed spinach in a
strainer and press firmly until
all of the liquid is removed and
the spinach is completely dry.
2. Combine the drained spinach with all of the remaining
ingredients in a mixing bowl
and mix thoroughly.
3. Refrigerate several hours or
overnight before serving.

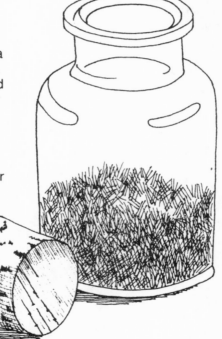

Dee Davis, a well-known fitness instructor in Phoenix,
Arizona, served a sensational
spinach spread as an hors
d'oeuvre one evening. It was
so delicious I asked her for
the recipe. Her recipe was far
too high in calories for my
book, so I told her I would
modify the recipe, reduce the
calories by at least two thirds
and send her my variation.
Here it is. This is a wonderful
salad, spread or dip. It can
even be used as a topping for
other cooked vegetables.

Makes 2 cups
1/4 cup contains approximately:
1/2 vegetable exchange
1 fat exchange
58 calories

VARIATION:

**STILL-LOWER-CALORIE SPINACH
SPREAD:** Substitute 1 cup of
Sauer Family Cream, page 42,
for the sour cream. Subtract 1
fat exchange and add 1/4 low-
fat meat exchange. This reduces the calories to 27 per
1/4 cup.

Make-Your-Own Yogurt

2 cups instant non-fat dry milk
1 gallon (4 quarts) non-fat milk
1 cup plain low-fat yogurt

1. Combine the dry and liquid non-fat milk in a large saucepan and mix thoroughly.
2. Heat slowly for 15 minutes over medium heat. *Do not boil.* Remove from the heat and allow to cool for 25 minutes. Skim off the film that forms on the surface.
3. Add the yogurt and mix well into the milk mixture.
4. Sterilize a large container (or containers) in boiling water. Pour the mixture into the sterilized container(s) for 3 to 6 hours. If you have a gas stove, place the container(s) in the oven and the pilot light will keep them at the proper temperature. If you do not have a gas stove, place the container(s) in warm water that you replace or replenish regularly to maintain the temperature.
5. When the mixture has thickened enough to hold together (test by tilting the container[s] slightly), refrigerate for 4 or 5 hours to thicken to the proper yogurt consistency.

This homemade yogurt can be used in any recipe calling for yogurt. If this is more yogurt than you can use in a week's time, reduce the recipe accordingly.

Makes 4 quarts
1 cup contains approximately:
1 non-fat milk exchange
80 calories

VARIATIONS:

VANILLA YOGURT: Add 1/2 cup fructose and 1/4 cup vanilla extract in step 3. Add 1/2 fruit exchange and 20 calories per cup. To make only 1 cup of vanilla yogurt, add 1-1/2 teaspoons fructose and 3/4 teaspoon vanilla extract to 1 cup of the prepared yogurt. This, too, will add 1/2 fruit exchange and 20 calories per cup. If you use 1 cup commercial low-fat yogurt, add exactly the same amount of fructose and vanilla extract. One cup will then contain approximately 1 low-fat milk exchange, 1/2 fruit exchange and 145 calories.

SALAD DRESSINGS AND SAUCES: June Biermann and Barbara Toohey have given me permission to quote these interesting yogurt flavor changes from their excellent book, *The Diabetic's Total Health Book:*

"Mustard Yogurt. Flavor the amount of non-fat yogurt you need for dressing with a bit of prepared mustard. We prefer Dijon, but any brand you like will serve the purpose.

"Oriental Yogurt. Add garlic powder and a small amount of soy sauce or tamari and ginger to the yogurt.

"Herbed Yogurt. Add any herbs you particularly like. One combination we favor is tarragon, basil and chervil. For an Italian touch, use oregano, basil and garlic. With spinach salad, try tarragon, garlic, a dash of artificial sweetener or fructose balanced off with a little vinegar to taste and artificial bacon bits.

"Minted Yogurt. Add a hint—but *just* a hint—of fresh mint. This is particularly good with fruit salads."

ALMOST RICOTTA CHEESE: Place a strainer over a large bowl and line it with two thicknesses of cheesecloth. Pour the prepared yogurt into the strainer. Using the edges of the cheesecloth, form a bag and press the liquid out into the bowl, adding weights if necessary. Let drain overnight in the refrigerator. Makes 5-1/2 cups. One-half cup contains approximately 1-1/2 non-fat milk exchanges and 120 calories.

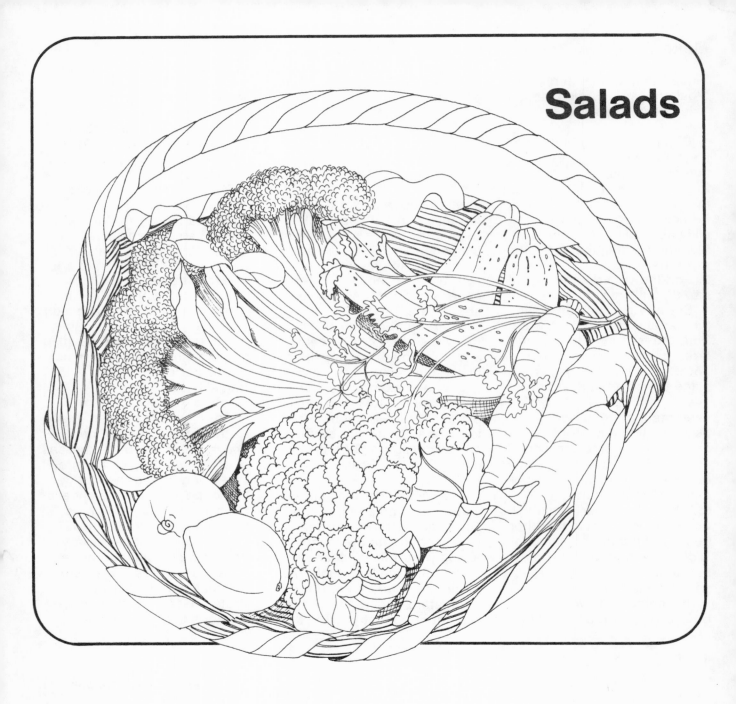

Salads

Salad Dressings

Many people believe that the way to lower calories is to eat salads most of the time. This is true only if you are using either very little salad dressing or a low-calorie one. Most salad dressings are so high in calories due to their fat content that a salad actually becomes a very high-calorie meal.

I developed the basic salad dressing series in this section for a menu program at the Canyon Ranch Vacation/Fitness Resort in Tucson, Arizona. These dressings are meant to duplicate the taste associated with classic oil-and-vinegar dressings, while greatly reducing the calories per serving. The Buttermilk Dressing series presented here provides a low-calorie, creamy dressing in a variety of flavor choices.

When dividing the salad-dressing recipe yields into smaller amounts for computing calories per serving, remember that there are 16 tablespoons in one cup of dressing.

Basic Dressing

1 teaspoon salt
1/4 cup red wine vinegar
1 teaspoon fructose
1/4 teaspoon freshly ground
  black pepper
1/4 teaspoon garlic powder
2 teaspoons fresh lemon juice
1 teaspoon Worcestershire
  sauce
1/4 teaspoon Dijon-style
  mustard
1/2 cup water
2 tablespoons corn oil

1. Dissolve the salt in the vinegar in a jar with a tightly fitting lid. Add all of the remaining ingredients, except the oil, and shake well.

2. Add the oil and shake vigorously for 1 full minute. Store in the refrigerator.

Makes 1 cup dressing
1 cup contains approximately:
1/2 fruit exchange
6 fat exchanges
290 calories
1 tablespoon contains approximately:
Exchanges negligible
18 calories

VARIATIONS:

ITALIAN DRESSING: Add 1-1/2 teaspoons crushed dried oregano, 1 teaspoon crushed dried basil and 1 teaspoon crushed dried tarragon before adding the oil.

CUMIN DRESSING: Add 1/4 teaspoon ground cumin before adding the oil.

TARRAGON DRESSING: Add 1-1/2 teaspoons crushed dried tarragon before adding the oil.

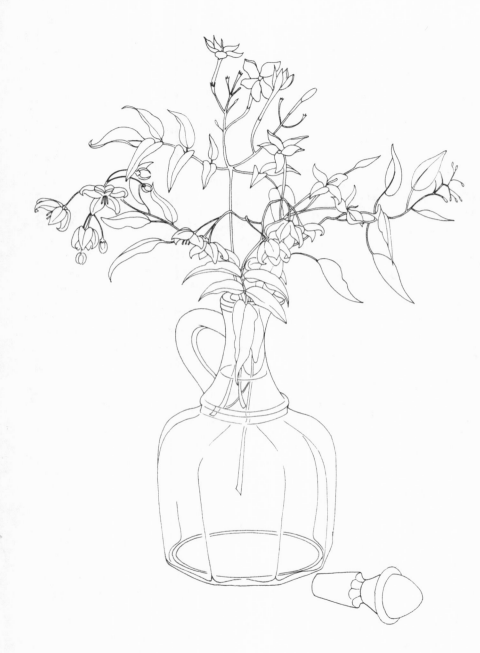

Buttermilk Dressing

2 tablespoons cornstarch
1 teaspoon dry mustard
1 teaspoon fructose
1/2 teaspoon seasoned salt
1/4 teaspoon garlic powder
Dash freshly ground black
    pepper
1/2 cup water
1 tablespoon corn oil
1 tablespoon cider vinegar
1/2 teaspoon Worcestershire
    sauce
1/2 cup buttermilk

1. Combine the cornstarch, mustard, fructose, seasoned salt, garlic powder and black pepper in a saucepan.
2. Add the water and mix thoroughly. Place over medium heat and cook, stirring constantly, until thickened.
3. Remove from the heat, add the corn oil and vinegar and mix thoroughly.
4. Slowly add the buttermilk, continuing to stir until smooth and creamy.

 This dressing will not hold for more than 2 days. When possible, make it the same day you plan to use it.

Makes 1-1/4 cups
1 tablespoon contains approximately:
1/4 fat exchange
12 calories

BARBECUE DRESSING: Add 1 teaspoon liquid smoke at the end of step 4.

MUSTARD SAUCE: Add 1 table-spoon prepared mustard at the end of step 4. This variation is best as a sauce on meats, hamburgers or hot dogs.

RED WINE VINEGAR DRESSING AND VARIATIONS: Substitute 1 tablespoon of red wine vinegar for the cider vinegar and use as is or use in one of the following variations.
● Blue Cheese Dressing: Add 1-1/4 ounces blue cheese, crumbled, at end of step 4; add 1-1/4 high-fat meat exchanges and 119 calories per 1-1/4 cups (add 6 calories per tablespoon).
● Stilton Dressing: Use Stilton cheese in place of blue cheese, above. Exchanges and calories are the same as for Blue Cheese Dressing.
● Parmesan Dressing: Use 1/4 cup grated Parmesan cheese in place of the blue cheese, above, and add 1 medium-fat meat exchange and 75 calories per 1-1/4 cups (add 4 calories per tablespoon).

LEMON-BUTTERMILK DRESSING AND VARIATIONS: Substitute 1 tablespoon of fresh lemon juice for the cider vinegar and use as is or use in one of the following variations.
● Horseradish Dressing: Add 1 teaspoon prepared horse-radish in step 1.
● Louie Dressing: Add 1-1/2 tablespoons tomato paste in step 1. Add 1/2 vegetable exchange and 13 calories per 1-1/4 cups (add 1 calorie per tablespoon).

Date-Cheese Dressing or Sauce

1 cup Date "Sugar," page 147
3/4 cup water
1 cup ricotta cheese or low-fat cottage cheese
1 teaspoon vanilla extract
1/4 teaspoon ground cinnamon

1. Combine the date "sugar" and water in a saucepan and bring to a boil over medium heat.

2. Reduce the heat and simmer, uncovered, for about 20 minutes, or until all of the liquid is absorbed.
3. Remove the pan from the heat and cool to room temperature. When cool, combine the date mixture with all of the remaining ingredients in a blender container and blend until smooth. Store, covered, in the refrigerator.

This is my favorite dressing on fruit salad. It is also good served with a turkey dinner in place of cranberry sauce.

Makes 2 cups
2 tablespoons contain approximately:
1/2 fruit exchange
1/4 low-fat meat exchange
34 calories

VARIATION:

POTASSIUM PINWHEELS: Following the directions for Banana-Peanut Pinwheels, page 148, substitute 2 tablespoons Date-Cheese Dressing for the peanut butter. One whole banana prepared this way contains 2-1/2 fruit exchanges and 1/4 low-fat meat exchange, a total of 114 calories. I call this variation Potassium Pinwheels because both dates and bananas are very high in potassium.

French Dressing Marinade

3 tablespoons red wine
  vinegar
1/2 teaspoon salt
2 tablespoons water
2 teaspoons fresh lemon juice
1/2 teaspoon dry mustard
1/2 teaspoon crushed dried
  basil
1/2 teaspoon celery seed
1/8 teaspoon freshly ground
  black pepper
1 garlic clove, crushed
2/3 cup corn oil

1. Combine the vinegar and
salt and stir until the salt is
dissolved.
2. Add all of the remaining
ingredients, except the oil, and
mix thoroughly.
3. Add the oil and mix thoroughly again. Pour the marinade into a jar with a tightly
fitting lid and shake vigorously
for 30 seconds. Store in the
refrigerator.

Makes 1 cup
1 tablespoon contains approximately:
2 fat exchanges
90 calories

VARIATION:

FRENCH SALAD DRESSING: Use
as a dressing on tossed salads.

Roquefort Dressing

1/2 cup crumbled Roquefort
  cheese
1 cup plain low-fat yogurt
1 garlic clove, minced
1/8 teaspoon freshly ground
  black pepper
1/2 teaspoon fresh lemon juice

1. Combine all of the ingredients and mix well.
2. Allow to stand at least 24
hours in the refrigerator before
using.
  Note: This dressing can be
further reduced in calories by
thinning it with non-fat milk.

Makes 1-1/2 cups dressing
1-1/2 cups contain approximately:
2 high-fat meat exchanges
1 low-fat milk exchange
315 calories
1 tablespoon contains approximately:
Exchanges negligible
13 calories

VARIATIONS:

BLUE CHEESE-YOGURT DRESSING:
Use blue cheese in place of the
Roquefort.

STILTON CHEESE DRESSING: Use
Stilton cheese in place of the
Roquefort.

Mandarin Dressing

1/4 cup sesame seeds
2/3 cup corn oil
2 tablespoons red wine vinegar
2 tablespoons fresh lemon
  juice
2 tablespoons soy sauce
2 tablespoons fructose
1 teaspoon garlic powder
1 tablespoon freshly grated
  ginger root, or
  1/2 teaspoon ground ginger

1. Preheat the oven to 350°F.
Place the sesame seeds on a
baking sheet in the center of
the preheated oven for 8 to 10
minutes, or until they are gold-
en brown. Watch them carefully, as they burn easily. Set
aside.
2. Combine all of the remaining
ingredients and mix well. Add
the toasted sesame seeds to
the dressing and pour into a
jar with a tightly fitting lid.
Shake vigorously for 1 full
minute.
3. Refrigerate for at least 24
hours before serving.
  This is not only a delicious
salad dressing, it is also an
excellent marinade for fish and
chicken. It is also a good
sauce for fruit, vegetables, fish,
poultry and meat.

Makes 1 cup dressing
1 tablespoon contains approximately:
2-1/2 fat exchanges
113 calories

VARIATION:

SHERRIED MANDARIN DRESSING:
Substitute 2 tablespoons of
sherry for the soy sauce. This
is a good variation for those
on sodium-restricted diets.

Low-Calorie Tomato Topping
(A Salad Dressing,
Sauce or Dip)

One 16-ounce can tomatoes,
   undrained
2 tablespoons fresh lemon juice
2 tablespoons red wine vinegar
1 teaspoon crushed dried
   oregano
1/2 teaspoon crushed dried
   basil
1/2 teaspoon crushed dried
   tarragon
1/4 teaspoon garlic powder
1/4 teaspoon onion powder
1/4 teaspoon freshly ground
   black pepper

1. Put all ingredients in a blender container and blend until
smooth. Store in the refrigerator.

Makes 2-1/2 cups
1/2 cup contains approximately:
1 vegetable exchange
25 calories

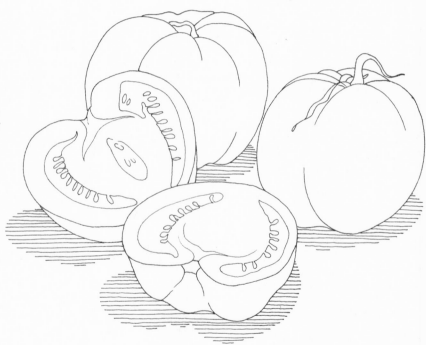

ITALIAN TUNA SALAD: Combine
the tomato topping with one
13-ounce can water-packed
tuna, drained and flaked, and
serve over shredded lettuce.
Makes 4 servings. Each serving contains approximately 2
low-fat meat exchanges, 1-1/4
vegetable exchanges and 142
calories.

Salads

Salads have great latitude in the diabetic diet because they can range from a small, practically calorie-free first course to a main course containing all of the necessary exchanges for a meal.

Always try to wash salad greens several hours before you plan to use them. Pat them dry, wrap them in towels and place in the refrigerator. Not only will your salads be crisper, but you will also need far less dressing to completely coat each leaf. When calories are precious, the less dressing the better.

Always serve your salads on very cold plates. It is a good idea, in fact, to chill your salad plates in the freezer.

Marinated Carrot Sticks

2 pounds (16 small) carrots, scraped and cut into slender sticks
1/2 cup tarragon vinegar
1/4 cup water
2 tablespoons fructose
1/2 teaspoon salt
Dash freshly ground black pepper
1 teaspoon crushed dried tarragon

1. Drop the carrot sticks into boiling water and cook until just tender, about 5 minutes. Drain well.

2. While the carrots are cooking, combine all of the remaining ingredients. Pour the mixture over the carrot sticks and allow them to cool to room temperature.

3. Store in the refrigerator in a non-metal container. Before packing the carrots for a picnic, drain them completely and put them in plastic bags or wrap in aluminum foil.

Makes 4 cups
1/2 cup contains approximately:
1 vegetable exchange
25 calories

VARIATION:

MARINATED GREEN BEANS: Substitute 2 pounds of green beans for the carrot sticks.

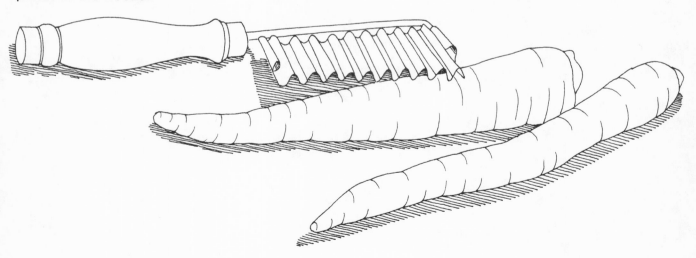

Eggplant Appetizer

1 large eggplant
1 onion, finely chopped
1 garlic clove, minced
1 large tomato, peeled and
  finely chopped
3/4 teaspoon salt
1/8 teaspoon freshly ground
  black pepper
2 teaspoons red wine vinegar
Sliced black olives for garnish
  (optional)

1. Preheat the oven to 400°F. Wash the eggplant and pierce the skin in several places.
2. Place the eggplant in a shallow pan and bake in the preheated oven until tender, about 30 minutes.
3. Allow the eggplant to cool until it can be easily handled, then peel it and chop into very small pieces.
4. Add all of the remaining ingredients to the eggplant and mix well.
5. Refrigerate the eggplant mixture until thoroughly chilled. Serve on lettuce leaves and garnish with sliced olives, if desired. (Remember that 5 small olives equal 1 fat exchange and 45 calories.)

This appetizer is even better if it is made the day before you plan to serve it.

Makes 8 servings
Each serving (without olive garnish)
  contains approximately:
1 vegetable exchange
25 calories

VARIATION:

EGGPLANT MARINARA: Add one 13-ounce can of water-packed tuna, drained and flaked, in step 3, and mix thoroughly. Chill well, then serve as described in the basic recipe. Add 1 low-fat meat exchange and 55 calories per serving.

Broccoli Vinaigrette

2 pounds broccoli spears
  (about 8 cups)
1 cup Basic Dressing, page 53
One 2-ounce jar sliced
  pimientos for garnish
1/4 cup capers for garnish

1. Steam the broccoli until tender but still crisp, about 5 minutes. Remove from the steamer and immediately place the broccoli under cold running water, then drain thoroughly.
2. Place the drained broccoli in a non-metal dish and pour the dressing over it. Cover and refrigerate all day or overnight.
3. To serve, remove the broccoli from the dressing and place on chilled plates. Garnish with pimiento strips and capers.

Makes 6 servings
Each serving contains approximately:
1 vegetable exchange
1 fat exchange
70 calories

VARIATIONS:

● Substitute any fresh vegetable in season for the broccoli. Follow the steaming directions on page 74 for cooking time and procedure. Check the vegetable exchange list for vegetable exchanges and calories per serving. Or try a combination of vegetables for a marinated vegetable medley. Marinated vegetables can be served as a first course in place of a salad. They are also excellent for a buffet, because they are more easily served than most salads.

CELERY VICTOR: Substitute whole stalks of celery heart, including the leaves, for the broccoli.

Taco Salad

1 head lettuce
1/2 pound ground beef sirloin
2 large tomatoes, diced
1-1/2 cups grated sharp
   cheddar cheese
3/4 cup Cumin Dressing,
   page 53
3 tablespoons sour cream
36 Toasted Tortilla Chips
   (1/2 recipe), page 140, for
   garnish

1. Wash and finely chop the lettuce. Place the lettuce in a colander so that the moisture can drip from the lettuce before preparing the salad. Place the colander in the refrigerator.
2. Crumble the ground sirloin in a cured iron skillet and cook over medium heat until just done.
3. Put the lettuce, tomatoes, cooked warm sirloin and 3/4 cup of the cheddar cheese in a large mixing bowl. Add the Cumin Dressing and toss well.
4. Divide the salad onto 6 plates. Sprinkle an equal amount of the remaining 3/4 cup of cheddar cheese evenly over each serving, then top each with 1-1/2 teaspoons of sour cream.

Garnish each serving with 6 Toasted Tortilla Chips.

Makes 6 servings
Each serving (with tortilla chips)
   contains approximately:
2 medium-fat meat exchanges
1 bread exchange
2 fat exchanges
310 calories

VARIATION:

CHICKEN TACO SALAD: Substitute 2 cups of diced cooked chicken for the beef and 1-1/2 cups of Monterey Jack cheese for the cheddar.

Tabbouli
(Lebanese Salad)

1 cup uncooked bulgur
   (cracked wheat)
1/4 cup fresh lemon juice
1/2 teaspoon salt
1/4 teaspoon freshly ground
   black pepper
1 garlic clove, minced
1 tablespoon water
2 tomatoes, finely diced
1 cup parsley sprigs, minced
1 cup chopped green onions
1/2 cup mint leaves, minced
36 small romaine lettuce leaves

1. Soak the bulgur in hot water to cover for 30 minutes.
2. While the bulgur is soaking, make the dressing. Combine the lemon juice and salt and stir until the salt is dissolved. Add the pepper, garlic and water and mix well. Put the dressing in a jar with a tightly fitting lid and shake vigorously for 30 seconds. Set aside.
3. Drain the bulgur thoroughly and place in a mixing bowl. Add the tomato, parsley, green onions, mint and dressing and toss well. Chill thoroughly.
4. Serve on chilled salad plates with each serving surrounded by 3 romaine leaves. Traditionally this salad is eaten by scooping it up on the romaine leaves.

   This tabbouli recipe differs from the one in *The Calculating Cook* in that it does not contain any olive oil. I have found that this one tastes just as good and eliminates the fat exchange and 45 calories per serving.

Makes 12 servings
Each serving contains approximately:
1 bread exchange
1/2 vegetable exchange
83 calories

VARIATIONS:

• Add 6 cups (3 pints) of low-fat cottage cheese in step 3 and mix thoroughly. Add 2 low-fat meat exchanges and 110 calories per serving.

• To make an hors-d'oeuvre spread from leftover tabbouli, add low-fat cottage cheese or drained and flaked water-packed tuna to taste (or a combination of the two). Check the low-fat meat exchange list for calorie and exchange adjustments.

• Add two 13-ounce cans of water-packed tuna, drained and flaked, in step 3, for a Mediterranean Medley Tuna Salad. Add 2 low-fat meat exchanges and 110 calories per serving.

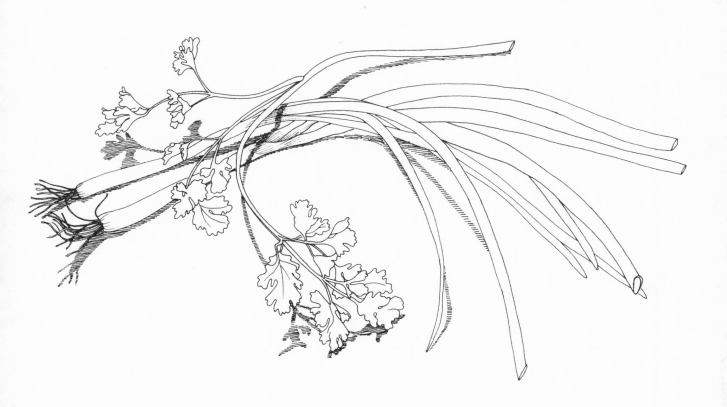

Candle Salad

4 cups shredded lettuce
8 asparagus spears
1 carrot, cooked
1 green bell pepper, seeded
  and cut into strips
1 red bell pepper, seeded
  and cut into strips

1. Divide the shredded lettuce evenly among 8 salad plates (1/2 cup on each plate).
2. Place 1 asparagus spear on top of the lettuce, simulating a candle. Place a small slice of cooked carrot, cut in the shape of a flame, on the top of each asparagus spear.
3. To make the candle holders, use strips of the red and green pepper alternately for the base. Use one curved strip of the pepper for the handle.

Makes 8 servings
Free food
Calories negligible

VARIATION: For a buffet, arrange all of the candles on a large platter.

Vegetable and Cottage Cheese Salad

2 cups (1 pint) low-fat
  cottage cheese
1 teaspoon freshly grated
  lemon rind
2 teaspoons fresh lemon juice
1 teaspoon crushed dried
  oregano
1/4 teaspoon freshly ground
  black pepper
2 cups broccoli flowerets,
  steamed and chilled
2 cups sliced (1/2 inch)
  zucchini, steamed and chilled
2 cups sliced (1/2 inch) yellow
  squash, steamed and chilled
2 carrots, cut in slender sticks,
  steamed and chilled
2 cups raw cauliflowerets,
  chilled
4 large parsley sprigs

1. Combine the cottage cheese, lemon rind, lemon juice, oregano and pepper and mix thoroughly.
2. Put 1/2 cup of the cottage cheese mixture in the center of each of 4 chilled plates. Arrange the vegetables attractively around the cottage cheese, alternating the colors. Garnish each serving with a parsley sprig.

Makes 4 servings
Each serving contains approximately:
2 vegetable exchanges
2 low-fat meat exchanges
160 calories

VARIATION: Any fresh vegetables may be substituted for those suggested. The more colorful the combination, the prettier the salad plate. Check the vegetable exchange list for exchange and calorie adjustments.

Fruit and Cottage Cheese Salad

2 cups (1 pint) low-fat
  cottage cheese
1 tablespoon freshly grated
  orange rind
1/2 teaspoon ground cinnamon
1 orange, peeled and thinly
  sliced
1 banana, thinly sliced
1 apple, unpeeled, cored and
  thinly sliced
1/2 cantaloupe, peeled,
  seeded and thinly sliced
1-1/2 cups whole fresh or
  frozen unsweetened strawberries, thawed, for garnish

1. Combine the cottage cheese, orange rind and cinnamon and mix well.
2. Put 1/2 cup of the cottage cheese mixture in the center of each of 4 chilled plates. Arrange the sliced fresh fruit attractively around the cottage cheese.
3. Garnish each plate with whole strawberries.

This fruit salad also makes a delicious breakfast, and a half portion is a good low-calorie dessert.

Makes 4 servings
Each serving contains approximately:
2 fruit exchanges
2 low-fat meat exchanges
190 calories

VARIATION: Any fresh fruit may be substituted for those suggested. Check the fruit exchange list for exchange and calorie adjustments.

Tomato and Mushroom Salad

3 tablespoons sunflower seeds
1/2 cup plain low-fat yogurt
1/2 garlic clove, minced, or
   1/8 teaspoon garlic powder
1/2 teaspoon fructose
1/2 teaspoon ground cumin
1/4 teaspoon salt
1 teaspoon fresh lemon juice
3 cups sliced mushrooms
   (3/4 pound)
1 large tomato, diced
6 lettuce leaves (optional)
6 parsley sprigs (optional)

1. Preheat the oven to 350°F. Place the sunflower seeds on a baking sheet in the center of the preheated oven for 8 to 10 minutes, or until a golden brown. Watch them carefully, as they burn easily. Set aside.
2. Combine the yogurt, garlic, fructose, cumin, salt and lemon juice and mix well.
3. Combine the yogurt mixture with the mushrooms and tomatoes and mix well.
4. Place a lettuce leaf on each of 6 salad plates, if desired. Divide the tomato-mushroom mixture evenly among the plates and garnish with parsley sprigs, if desired.
5. Sprinkle 1-1/2 teaspoons of the sunflower seeds over the top of each serving.

Makes 6 servings
Each serving contains approximately:
1 vegetable exchange
1 fat exchange
60 calories

VARIATIONS:
● Add 1-1/2 cups grated Monterey Jack cheese in step 3. Add 1 high-fat meat exchange and 95 calories per serving.
● Add two 6-ounce cans of water-packed tuna, drained and flaked, in step 3. Add 3/4 low-fat meat exchange and 41 calories per serving.
● Add 4 hard-cooked eggs, chopped, to the salad in step 3. Add 3/4 medium-fat meat exchange and 57 calories per serving.

Gazpacho Salad

2 envelopes (2 tablespoons)
　unflavored gelatin
4 cups (1 quart) tomato juice
1/2 cup boiling water
2 teaspoons Worcestershire
　sauce
1 drop Tabasco sauce
3/4 teaspoon seasoned salt
1/4 teaspoon garlic powder
1/2 onion, finely chopped
1 small green bell pepper,
　seeded and finely chopped
1/2 large cucumber, peeled
　and finely chopped
1 large tomato, finely chopped
2 green onions, finely chopped
2 canned green chili peppers,
　seeded and finely chopped
2 lemons, cut into wedges, for
　garnish (optional)
8 parsley sprigs for garnish
　(optional)

1. Soften the gelatin in 1/4
cup of the tomato juice for 5
minutes. Add the boiling water
and stir until the gelatin is
completely dissolved.
2. Add the remaining tomato
juice, Worcestershire sauce,
Tabasco sauce, seasoned salt
and garlic powder and mix
well.
3. Add all of the remaining
ingredients, except the garnishes, and again mix thoroughly.
4. Pour into an oiled 8-cup
mold and refrigerate until firm
before serving.
5. Serve on chilled plates and
garnish with lemon wedges
and parsley sprigs.
　Serve this salad with Toasted
Tortilla Chips, if desired.

Makes 8 servings
Each serving contains approximately:
1 vegetable exchange
25 calories

VARIATIONS:

CHICKEN GAZPACHO SALAD: Add
2 cups chopped cooked chicken
and serve 4 people instead of
8. Add 1 vegetable exchange,
2 low-fat meat exchanges and
135 calories per serving.

CLASSIC GAZPACHO: Omit the
gelatin and boiling water and
all of step 1. Put 2 cups of the
tomato juice in a blender container with all of the remaining
ingredients, except the garnishes, and blend until smooth.
Add the remaining tomato juice
and again mix thoroughly. Serve
in chilled bowls, garnished with
lemon wedges and parsley sprigs.
Makes 8 servings. Each serving
contains approximately 1 vegetable exchange and 25 calories.

Artichoke Salad Plate

1 large artichoke
Vinegar
1/2 teaspoon salt
1 bay leaf
1/4 cup Curry Dip, page 42

1. Place the artichoke in a
saucepan with water to cover.
Add 1 tablespoon of vinegar
per quart of water. Add the
salt and bay leaf and bring to
a boil.
2. Reduce the heat, cover and
simmer the artichoke for approximately 30 minutes, or until
a leaf pulls away easily and
the base can be easily pierced
with a fork.
3. Remove the artichoke from
the water and cool to room
temperature.
4. Remove all of the leaves
from the artichoke, reserving
them, and scoop all of the
furry choke part from the heart.
This is done most easily with a
serrated grapefruit spoon.
5. Place the heart in the center
of a large plate and cut into
bite-sized pieces.
6. Arrange the leaves around
the heart in a flowerlike design.
7. Serve with Curry Dip as an
hors d'oeuvre, or place a small
amount of dip (total of 1/4
cup) on each leaf before arrang-
ing them around the heart.

Artichoke salad plates make excellent buffet salads and hors d'oeuvres.

Each artichoke (with dip) contains
 approximately:
1 vegetable exchange (depending
 upon the size of the artichoke)
1 low-fat meat exchange
80 calories

VARIATION: Substitute Clam Dip, page 42, for the Curry Dip. Add 1-1/2 low-fat meat exchanges and 83 calories per serving.

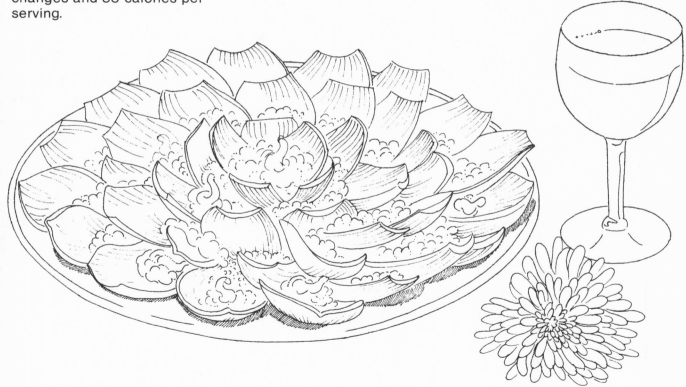

Zucchini Mousse

3 cups cooked chopped
   zucchini
2 envelopes (2 tablespoons)
   unflavored gelatin
1/4 cup cold water
1/2 cup boiling water
1/2 teapoon salt
Dash freshly ground black
   pepper
2 teaspoons Worcestershire
   sauce
1/2 cup evaporated skim milk,
   chilled

1. Put the cooked zucchini into a blender container and blend until completely puréed. Set aside.
2. Soften the gelatin in the cold water for 5 minutes. Add the boiling water and stir until the gelatin is completely dissolved.
3. Combine the puréed zucchini and gelatin mixtures, salt, pepper and Worcestershire sauce and mix well. Refrigerate for 30 minutes, or until slightly thickened.
4. Beat the chilled evaporated milk until it is at least 4 times its original volume.

5. Fold the whipped milk into the zucchini mixture, continuing to fold until no streaks of white show.
6. Pour into an oiled 6-cup mold and chill until set.

Makes 8 servings
Each serving contains approximately:
Exchanges negligible
20 calories

VARIATIONS:
● Use 3 cups of any cooked vegetable you choose in place of the zucchini. Check the vegetable exchange list for exchange and calorie adjustments.
● Add 2 tablespoons of Dill Sauce, page 44, to each serving. Add 2 fat exchanges and 90 calories per serving.

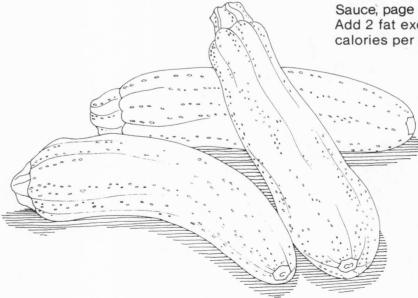

Tomato Aspic

4 cups (1 quart) tomato juice
1/4 cup finely chopped onion
1 bay leaf
1/8 teaspoon ground cloves
1/4 teaspoon freshly ground
    black pepper
1 teaspoon celery seed
1 teaspoon salt
2 envelopes (2 tablespoons)
    unflavored gelatin
1/4 cup cold water
1 tablespoon fresh lemon juice
One 8-ounce can crushed
    pineapple packed in natural
    juice, undrained

1. Combine the tomato juice,
onion, bay leaf, cloves, pepper,
celery seed and salt in a large
saucepan.
2. Bring to a boil, reduce the
heat and simmer, covered, for
20 minutes.
3. Remove from the heat, remove the bay leaf and set the
juice aside.
4. Soften the gelatin in the
cold water for 5 minutes. Add
the softened gelatin and the
lemon juice to the hot tomato
juice mixture and stir until the
gelatin is completely dissolved.
5. Allow the aspic to come to
room temperature and start to
jell slightly.

6. Add the can of pineapple
and all of the juice from the
can and mix thoroughly.
7. Pour the aspic into an oiled
6-cup mold and chill until firm.
   Make this aspic in a ring
mold for buffet luncheons and
fill the center with a fish, poultry or meat salad.

Makes 8 servings
Each serving contains approximately:
1/4 fruit exchange
1 vegetable exchange
35 calories

VARIATION:

TOMATO-TURKEY ASPIC: Add 2
cups of chopped cooked turkey when adding the pineapple.
Add 1 low-fat meat exchange
and 55 calories per serving.

Jelled Vegetable Salad

1 envelope (1 tablespoon)
    unflavored gelatin
2 tablepoons cold water
1/4 cup boiling water
1-3/4 cups chicken stock
1/2 cup cooked thinly sliced
    carrots
1 cup cooked cauliflowerets
1/2 cup cooked thinly sliced
    zucchini
1/2 red bell pepper, seeded
    and thinly sliced (if unavail-
    able, use green bell pepper)

1. Soften the gelatin in the
cold water for 5 minutes. Add
the boiling water and stir until
the gelatin is completely dissolved.
2. Combine the water-gelatin
mixture and the chicken stock
and mix well.
3. Chill, stirring occasionally,
until the mixture is the consistency of beaten egg whites.
4. Fold in all of the vegetables
and put in an oiled 4-cup
mold. Chill until set.
   This vegetable salad is excellent with Dill Sauce, page 44,
spooned over the top.

Makes 8 servings
Each serving contains approximately:
1/2 vegetable exchange
13 calories

VARIATION: This salad may
be made with any combination
of cooked frozen or fresh vegetables totaling 2 cups. This is
a marvelous way to use leftover cooked vegetables. Check
the vegetable exchange list
for exchanges and calories
per serving.

Jelled Fruit Salad

1 envelope (1 tablespoon)
  unflavored gelatin
2 tablespoons cold water
1/4 cup boiling water
1-2/3 cups unsweetened apple
  juice
1 cup thinly sliced fresh
  peaches or canned water-
  packed peaches, drained
1 small banana, peeled and
  sliced

1. Soften the gelatin in the cold water for 5 minutes. Add the boiling water and stir until the gelatin is completely dissolved.
2. Combine the water-gelatin mixture and the apple juice and mix well.
3. Chill, stirring occasionally, until the mixture is the consistency of beaten egg whites.
4. Fold in the sliced fruit and put in an oiled 4-cup mold. Chill until set.

Makes 8 servings
Each serving contains approximately:
1-1/4 fruit exchanges
50 calories

VARIATION: This fruit salad can be made with any combination of 2 cups of chopped or sliced fresh fruits or canned unsweetened fruits, drained. Check the fruit exchange list for exchange and calorie adjustments.

Cranberry-Apple Holiday Wreath Salad

4 large (or 6 small) apples,
  peeled, cored and diced
1-1/2 tablespoons fresh
  lemon juice
4 cups water
1/2 cup fructose
1 teaspoon ground cinnamon
1-1/2 tablespoons vanilla
  extract
1 pound (4 cups) fresh or
  frozen unsweetened
  cranberries
2 envelopes (2 tablespoons)
  unflavored gelatin
1/2 cup boiling water
1-1/2 cups non-fat milk
1/2 cup low-fat plain yogurt
1/2 cup dry white wine
  (preferably Chablis)
Watercress or parsley sprigs
  for garnish

1. Sprinkle the diced apples with the lemon juice and set aside.

2. In a large saucepan, combine the water, fructose, cinnamon and vanilla. Bring the mixture to a boil. Reduce the heat and simmer for 5 minutes. Add the cranberries to the simmering liquid and cook for 10 minutes. Add the apples to the cranberries and cook together for 10 more minutes.
3. Remove from the heat and cool to room temperature. Refrigerate until cold. If possible, allow the cranberries and apples to marinate overnight in the poaching liquid.
4. Remove the cranberry-apple mixture from the refrigerator and drain off the poaching liquid, reserving 1/2 cup of this liquid. Add the gelatin to the 1/2 cup cold poaching liquid and allow it to soften for at least 5 minutes. Add 1/2 cup boiling water to the gelatin mixture and stir until the gelatin is completely dissolved.
5. Put the cranberry-apple mixture into the blender container. Add the poaching liquid and as much of the milk as is necessary to purée the cranberries and apples. When the mixture is a liquid consistency,

pour it into a large mixing bowl and add the remaining milk and the yogurt and white wine. Mix thoroughly, using a wire whisk.

6. Pour the mixture into a 12-cup oiled ring mold. Chill for several hours or, preferably, overnight before unmolding. To unmold, tap the bottom and sides of the mold with the handle of a knife. Place a large plate over the mold and invert quickly.

7. Garnish with watercress or parsley sprigs for a touch of holiday greenery. This makes a beautiful and colorful holiday salad.

Makes 12 servings
Each serving contains approximately:
1-1/4 fruit exchanges
50 calories

VARIATION:

CRANBERRY-APPLE-NUT HOLIDAY WREATH SALAD: Sprinkle 3/4 cup of chopped toasted walnuts evenly over the top of the unmolded salad before serving. I also like to add a touch of Whipped "Cream," page 43, to each serving. Add 1/2 fat exchange and 23 calories per serving.

Tuna Salad in Cantaloupe Bowls

2 tablespoons raw sunflower seeds
2 small ripe cantaloupes
One 13-ounce can water-packed tuna, drained and flaked
1/4 cup finely chopped chives or green onion tops
1/2 teaspoon curry powder
4 parsley sprigs for garnish

1. Preheat the oven to 350°F. Place the sunflower seeds on a baking sheet in the center of the preheated oven for 8 to 10 minutes, or until a golden brown. Watch them carefully, as they burn easily. Set aside.
2. Cut the cantaloupes in half in a sawtooth pattern. Remove the seeds and then, using a melon baller, remove the cantaloupe pulp, being careful not to cut through the outer shell.
3. Combine the melon balls and all of the remaining ingredients, except the parsley sprigs, in a mixing bowl and mix well.
4. Divide the mixture evenly among the 4 cantaloupe bowls. Garnish each with a parsley sprig.

Makes 4 servings
Each serving contains approximately:
1 fat exchange
2 fruit exchanges
2 low-fat meat exchanges
235 calories

VARIATIONS:

TUNA IN CANTALOUPE BASKETS: Using 4 cantaloupes, draw the basket shape you wish on the outside of each cantaloupe, then carefully cut the cantaloupe to form the basket. Remove all of the cantaloupe pulp, using a melon baller. Use only *half* of the cantaloupe pulp and mix with the other ingredients as described in step 3. Use the remaining cantaloupe pulp for another purpose.

SHRIMP IN CANTALOUPE BOWLS: Substitute 2 cups of cooked shrimp for the tuna.

CHICKEN OR TURKEY IN CANTALOUPE BOWLS: Substitute 2 cups of chopped cooked chicken or turkey for the tuna.

Dilled Salmon Salad

Two 7-ounce cans salmon,
  drained and flaked
1 tablespoon fresh lemon juice
Dash cayenne pepper
2 tablespoons finely chopped
  fresh dill, or 1 teaspoon
  crushed dried dill weed
Lettuce leaves or shredded
  lettuce
Celery sticks for garnish
  (optional)
Cherry tomatoes for garnish
  (optional)
Capers for garnish (optional)

1. Combine the salmon, lemon juice, cayenne pepper and dill and toss thoroughly.
2. Line 4 salad plates with the lettuce leaves or shredded lettuce. Divide the salmon evenly among the 4 plates. Garnish each serving with celery sticks, cherry tomatoes and/or capers, if desired. Serve either with Mock Mayonnaise or Dill Sauce.

Makes 4 servings
Each serving (without dressing) con-
  approximately:
2 low-fat meat exchanges
110 calories

VARIATION:

DILLED TUNA SALAD: Substitute two 7-ounce cans water-packed tuna for the salmon.

Chicken Chop Suey Salad

2 celery stalks without leaves,
  sliced
1 green bell pepper, seeded
  and thinly sliced
2 onions, thinly sliced
2 cups thinly sliced fresh
  mushrooms (1/2 pound), or
  two 8-ounce cans sliced
  mushrooms, drained
One 10-ounce package frozen
  Chinese pea pods, thawed
One 16-ounce can sliced
  bamboo shoots, drained
One 16-ounce can water
  chestnuts, drained and sliced
1/2 cup soy sauce
1/2 teaspoon freshly ground
  black pepper
1 tablespoon Worcestershire
  sauce
4 cups julienne-cut skinned
  cooked chicken

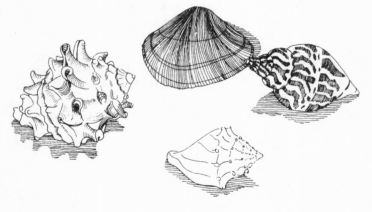

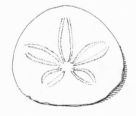

1. Half fill a large saucepan with water and bring to a rapid boil.

2. Put the celery, green pepper, onions and fresh mushrooms (if you are using them) into the boiling water. Allow the water to return to a rapid boil and immediately remove from the heat. Drain the vegetables well in a colander or strainer. Run cold water over the vegetables and drain thoroughly. Refrigerate until chilled.

3. Combine the chilled vegetables with the thawed pea pods, bamboo shoots and water chestnuts in a large bowl. (If you are using canned mushrooms, add them now.)

4. Combine the soy sauce, black pepper and Worcestershire sauce and mix well.

5. Combine the sliced chicken and the vegetables, then pour the dressing over the top and toss thoroughly. Serve on chilled plates.

Serve this salad with a side dish of cold cooked rice and use chopsticks as utensils, if you like.

Makes 8 servings
Each serving contains approximately:
2 vegetable exchanges
2 low-fat meat exchanges
160 calories

VARIATIONS:

• Substitute cooked shrimp or any cold julienne-cut cooked *lean* meat of choice for the chicken. Even water-packed tuna, drained and flaked, is good.

• Omit the meat and serve as a vegetarian dish. Omit the low-fat meat exchanges and subtract 110 calories per serving.

Hot Dog Salad

6 all-beef weiners
2 cups well-drained sauerkraut
1/2 cup finely chopped carrots
1 cup finely chopped celery
1 cup finely chopped green
  bell pepper
1 cup finely chopped red bell
  pepper
1/2 cup finely chopped onion
1/4 cup white vinegar
1/4 cup fructose
1/8 teaspoon freshly ground
  black pepper
1 cup Herbed Mustard,
  page 44
Parsley sprigs for garnish
Sliced tomatoes for garnish

1. Slice each weiner in half lengthwise and place the halves under a broiler until lightly browned on both sides.

2. Remove from the broiler and cool to room temperature. Chop the broiled weiners into small pieces and set aside.

3. Put the sauerkraut in a colander and rinse with cold water. Allow to drain thoroughly.

4. Combine the drained sauerkraut, chopped weiners and all the remaining ingredients, except the Herbed Mustard and garnishes, and mix thoroughly. Serve with Herbed Mustard and garnish with parsley sprigs and tomato slices.

Makes 6 servings
Each serving contains approximately:
2 vegetable exchanges
1 high-fat meat exchange
3/4 fruit exchange
175 calories

SAUERKRAUT SALAD: Omit the weiners and subtract 1 high-fat meat exchange and 95 calories per serving.

Vegetables

Vegetables

Steaming vegetables for people who have never seen it done properly is always fun for me. It is a great "show and tell," because your audience will see rather mundane-looking raw vegetables become gorgeous and brightly colored right before their eyes, and usually in just two to three minutes. The color and texture of the vegetables are then preserved by running them under cold water whether they are going to be served cold or reheated to be served hot. Not only are these vegetables beautiful in appearance, but they are also wonderful to eat.

I have had people tell me they do not like to cook vegetables like broccoli, cauliflower or cabbage in their own homes because of the strong smell they produce when they're cooking. My home is never filled with these unpleasant odors, because once you can *smell* a vegetable cooking, you have overcooked it.

Directions for Steaming Vegetables

When steaming vegetables, always make certain that the steamer basket is above the level of the water and that the water is boiling rapidly before the vegetables are covered and timing is begun.

Once the vegetables have steamed for the correct length of time, immediately place them under cold running water. This stops the cooking quickly and preserves both their color and texture.

When reheating vegetables prepared in this manner, be careful not to overcook them in the reheating process or they will lose both their crispness and their color.

Whether you are going to be serving vegetables hot or cold, they can be prepared in advance and stored, covered, in the refrigerator. Many of the recipes in this section call for steamed vegetables, and by being able to prepare them in advance, preparation at meal time can be greatly shortened.

In the following steaming chart, the time given for steaming each vegetable produces a tender yet crisp result. Mushy, colorless vegetables are not only tasteless, but have been robbed of much of their nutritional value by overcooking.

Fresh Vegetable Steaming Chart

Vegetable	Minutes	Vegetable	Minutes	Vegetable	Minutes
Asparagus	5	Collards	1-2	Pea pods	3
Beans:		Corn:		Peas	3-5
green	5	kernels	3	Peppers:	
lima	5	on the cob	3	chili	2-3
string or snap	5	Coriander (cilantro)	1-2	green and red bell	2
Bean sprouts	1-2	Cucumber	2-3	Pimientos	2
Beet greens	3-5	Dandelion greens	1-2	Poke	3
Beets, quartered	15	Eggplant, cut up	5	Potatoes:	
Black radish,		Garlic	5	sweet, ½-inch slices	15
½-inch slices	5	Jerusalem artichokes	8	white, ½-inch slices	10
Breadfruit	10	Jicama	10	Pumpkin, cut up	5
Broccoli:		Kale	1-2	Radishes	5
flowerets	3-5	Kohlrabi, quartered	8-10	Rhubarb	5
branches	5	Leeks	5	Romaine lettuce	1-2
Brussels sprouts	5	Lettuce	1-2	Rutabagas	8
Cabbage, quartered	5	Lotus root,		Shallots	2
Carrots, ½-inch slices	5	¼-inch slices	25	Spinach	1-2
Cauliflower:		Mint	1-2	Squash:	
flowerets	3	Mushrooms	2	acorn, cut up	5
whole	5	Mustard, fresh	1-2	hubbard, cut up	5
Celery root	3-4	Okra	5	summer	3
Celery stalks	10	Onions:		zucchini	3
Chard	1-2	green tops	3	Tomatoes	3
Chayote	3	whole	5	Turnips, quartered	8
Chicory	1-2	Palm hearts	5	Water chestnuts	8
Chives	2-3	Parsley	1-2	Watercress	1-2

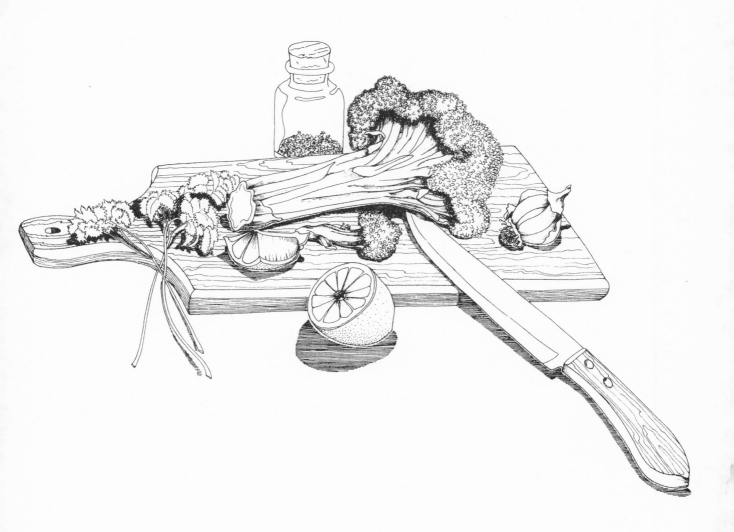

Herbed Vegetable Medley

4 cups assorted vegetables from preceding chart
2 tablespoons corn oil margarine
1/4 teaspoon salt
1 teaspoon crushed dried basil
1/4 cup finely chopped parsley
1/4 cup finely chopped chives or green onion tops

1. Steam the vegetables according to the preceding chart, until tender but still crisp. Rinse vegetables under cold running water. Drain and set aside.
2. Melt the margarine in a large skillet. Add the salt, basil, parsley and chives.
3. Add the cooked vegetables to the skillet and mix thoroughly. Heat just to serving temperature.

Makes 8 servings
Each serving contains approximately:
1/2 vegetable exchange
3/4 fat exchange
47 calories

VARIATIONS:

HERBED CARROTS AND PARSLEY: Follow the basic recipe, using 8 thinly sliced carrots instead of the vegetable mixture. Omit the chives and use 1/2 cup of minced parsley.

LOW-CALORIE VEGETABLE MEDLEY Substitute 1/2 cup chicken stock for the margarine. Subtract 1 fat exchange and 45 calories per serving.

Vegetables with Curried Vegetable Dip

Curried Vegetable Dip
1 large head cauliflower, broken into flowerets
1 medium onion, finely chopped
3/4 teaspoon salt
1/8 teaspoon white pepper
1/2 cup water
1 cup low-fat milk
2 teaspoons corn oil margarine
1 tablespoon all-purpose flour
1 teaspoon curry powder
1/4 teaspoon ground ginger
1/4 teaspoon Worcestershire sauce
1 teaspoon fresh lemon juice

Suggested Raw Vegetables
Cauliflowerets
Celery sticks
Broccoli, cut into small pieces
Lettuce leaves, rolled
Radishes

1. To prepare the dip, place the cauliflowerets in a large saucepan with a lid. Add the onion, salt, pepper and water and bring to a boil.
2. Reduce the heat and simmer, covered, until fork-tender, about 15 to 20 minutes.
3. Put the cooked cauliflower and its cooking liquid in a blender container and blend until smooth and creamy. Set aside.
4. Put the milk in a saucepan and place over low heat.
5. In another saucepan, melt the margarine and add the flour, stirring constantly. Cook, stirring, for 3 minutes. *Do not brown.*

6. Take the flour-margarine mixture off the heat and add the simmering milk all at once, stirring constantly with a wire whisk.
7. Put the white sauce back on low heat and cook for 20 minutes, stirring occasionally.
8. Remove the sauce from the heat and add the cauliflower-onion mixture and all of the remaining ingredients.
9. Cool to room temperature and refrigerate until chilled before serving. Serve with the suggested vegetables or any vegetables of choice.

Makes 8 (1/2 cup) servings
Each serving contains approximately:
1 vegetable exchange
1/4 fat exchange
37 calories

VARIATION:

VEGETABLES WITH HORSERADISH DIP: Omit the curry and ginger from the dip and add 1 tablespoon of prepared horseradish and 1 additional teaspoon of Worcestershire sauce.

Minted Peas

2 cups fresh or frozen peas
1 teaspoon arrowroot
1/4 cup water
1 teaspoon fructose
4 teaspoons corn oil margarine
1/4 teaspoon salt
1/2 cup minced fresh mint leaves

1. Steam the peas until tender but still crisp, about 2 minutes. Be careful not to overcook them. Set aside in a bowl.
2. Dissolve the arrowroot in water in a saucepan, add the fructose and cook, stirring constantly, over medium heat until the mixture comes to a boil. Simmer, stirring, until clear and thickened, about 2 minutes.
3. Remove from the heat and add the margarine and salt, then pour over the steamed peas.
4. Add the mint and toss, mixing the ingredients thoroughly.

Makes 8 servings
Each serving contains approximately:
1 vegetable exchange
1/2 fat exchange
48 calories

VARIATION:

MINTED CARROTS: Substitute carrots for the peas. Subtract 1/2 vegetable exchange and 13 calories per serving.

Spicy Beets

1-1/2 cups diced or julienne-cut cooked beets, or one 16-ounce can diced or julienne-cut beets, drained
1/2 teaspoon fructose
1/2 teaspoon salt
1/8 teaspoon freshly ground black pepper
1 teaspoon onion powder
1 teaspoon prepared horseradish
2 teaspoons cider vinegar

1. Combine all of the ingredients and mix thoroughly.
2. Serve hot or cold as a vegetable side dish or salad.
   This is best if made 1 or 2 days before you plan to use it. Store it, covered, in the refrigerator.

Makes 6 (1/4 cup) servings
Each serving contains approximately:
1/2 vegetable exchange
13 calories

BEET RELISH: Chop the beets very finely and add 1 additional tablespoon of prepared horseradish. This is an excellent low-calorie relish with cold meat or poultry.

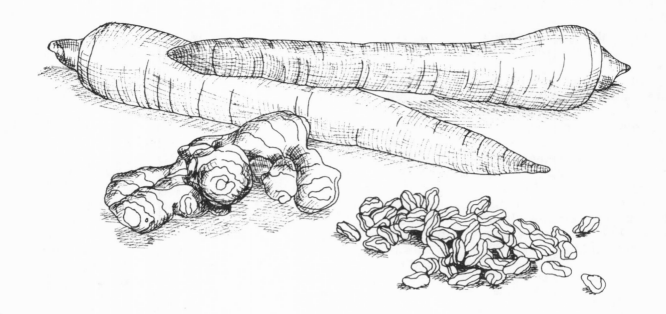

Curried Carrots and Raisins

2 tablespoons corn oil
  margarine
1/4 teaspoon salt
1 teaspoon curry powder
1 tablespoon freshly grated
  ginger root, or 1/2 teaspoon
  ground ginger
6 medium carrots, scraped
  and grated (3 cups)
1/4 cup finely chopped chives
  or green onion tops
1/2 cup raisins

1. Melt the margarine in a skillet. Add the salt, curry powder and ginger and mix thoroughly.
2. Add the carrots, chives and raisins and cook, stirring constantly, until carrots are tender but still crisp, about 5 minutes.

Makes 6 servings
Each serving contains approximately:
1 fat exchange
1 vegetable exchange
3/4 fruit exchange
100 calories

VARIATIONS:

● Serve cold as a salad.

CURRIED CARROTS AND RAISINS WITH CHEESE: Put 3 cups of low-fat cottage cheese in the bottom of a 3-quart casserole. Put the cooked Curried Carrots and Raisins over the top. (Or place 1/2 cup cottage cheese in the bottom of each of 6 au gratin dishes and put 1/2 cup of the carrots and raisins on top of each serving.) Place in a preheated 350°F oven for 10 minutes or until the cottage cheese is hot. Add 2 low-fat meat exchanges and 110 calories per serving.

Gingered Bean Sprouts

1 tablespoon corn oil
1 tablespoon freshly grated ginger root, or 1/4 teaspoon ground ginger
4 cups (3/4 pound) bean sprouts, washed, thoroughly drained and completely dried
1 tablespoon soy sauce

1. Heat the corn oil in a large skillet. Add the ginger and mix thoroughly.
2. Add the bean sprouts and stir-fry until the oil coats all of the sprouts.
3. Sprinkle the soy sauce over the bean sprouts. Toss thoroughly and serve at once.

Makes 4 servings
Each serving contains approximately:
1 vegetable exchange
3/4 fat exchange
59 calories

VARIATIONS:

• Substitute alfalfa sprouts for the bean sprouts.
• Add 2 cups julienne-cut cooked lean meat or poultry in step 2. Add 2 low-fat meat exchanges and 110 calories per serving.

COLD GINGERED BEAN SPROUTS AND VARIATION: Cool Gingered Bean Sprouts to room temperature. Refrigerate until cold and serve as a vegetable side dish or salad.
• Add 2 cups julienne-cut cooked turkey, chicken or shrimp and one 8-ounce can pineapple chunks packed in natural juice, drained, to Cold Gingered Bean Sprouts and serve as an entrée. Add 2 low-fat meat exchanges, 1/2 fruit exchange and 130 calories per serving.

Vegetable Dressing

1/2 cup almonds, finely chopped
2 eggs, lightly beaten, or 1/2 cup liquid egg substitute
1 teaspoon crushed dried marjoram or rosemary
1 teaspoon crushed dried oregano
1 teaspoon crushed dried sage
1/2 teaspoon crushed dried thyme
1/4 teaspoon salt
1 medium eggplant, unpeeled and diced
2 large onions, finely chopped
2 large red apples, unpared and diced
1 cup finely chopped parsley

1. Preheat the oven to 350°F. Place the finely chopped almonds on a baking sheet in the center of the preheated oven for 8 to 10 minutes, or until a golden brown. Watch them carefully, as they burn easily. Set aside. Leave the oven set at 350°F.
2. Combine the beaten eggs, marjoram, oregano, sage, thyme and salt in a large bowl and mix thoroughly.
3. Add all of the remaining ingredients, except the almonds, to the egg mixture and again mix thoroughly.
4. Transfer to a casserole, cover and bake for 1 hour in the preheated oven.
5. Before serving, mix the toasted almonds into the dressing, or sprinkle an equal amount of almonds over the top of each serving.

Makes 8 servings
Each serving contains approximately:
1 vegetable exchange
1/4 medium-fat meat exchange
3/4 fat exchange
1/4 fruit exchange
88 calories

VARIATION:

VEGETABLE DRESSING AU GRATIN: Just before serving, sprinkle 1 cup grated Monterey Jack cheese over the casserole and place under the broiler until the cheese is melted. Add 1/2 high-fat meat exchange and 48 calories per serving.

Indian Corn Stew

1 cup water
1/2 teaspoon salt
1/2 teaspoon chili powder
1/4 teaspoon freshly ground
   black pepper
2 cups fresh corn kernels (3
   ears of corn) or frozen corn
   kernels
1 onion, sliced
2 garlic cloves, minced
3 zucchini, cut into 1/4-inch-
   thick slices
2 large tomatoes, quartered
   and sliced
1 cup grated or crumbled
   sharp cheddar cheese
   (4 ounces)

1. Combine the water, salt, chili powder and pepper in a large saucepan and mix well.
2. Add the corn kernels, onion and garlic, place over medium heat and bring to a boil.
3. Reduce the heat, cover and simmer for 5 minutes.
4. Add the zucchini and cook for another 5 minutes. Add the tomatoes and cook until the tomatoes are warm but not mushy.
5. Add the cheese, mix well and heat just until melted.

Makes 6 servings
Each serving contains approximately:
1 bread exchange
1 vegetable exchange
3/4 high-fat meat exchange
167 calories

VARIATIONS:
● Substitute Monterey Jack cheese for the cheddar cheese.
● Add 2 cups of diced cooked lean meat or poultry for a main course when adding the tomatoes. Add 1-1/4 low-fat meat exchanges and 69 calories per serving.
● Omit the cheese for a lower-calorie vegetable side dish. Subtract 3/4 high-fat meat exchange and 72 calories per serving.

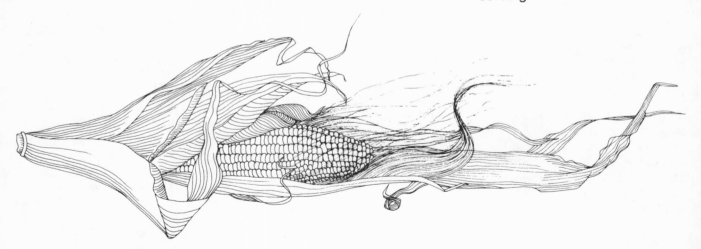

Cheesy Cauliflower

1 tablespoon corn oil
3 garlic cloves, chopped
2 teaspoons crushed dried
  basil
1 small cauliflower, broken
  into small flowerets
1/2 teaspoon salt
1/2 teaspoon freshly ground
  black pepper
One 16-ounce can tomato
  sauce
1/2 cup shredded cheddar
  cheese
1 cup hot cooked white rice
1/4 cup grated Parmesan
  cheese

1. Heat the oil in a large skillet.
Add the garlic and basil and
sauté for 2 minutes.
2. Add the cauliflower, salt and
pepper and sauté until tender
but still crisp.
3. Add the tomato sauce and
mix thoroughly. Reduce the
heat and simmer, uncovered,
for 20 minutes, stirring occasionally.
4. Combine the cheddar cheese
and the hot rice and toss
lightly. Place on a large platter
or on individual plates.
5. Pour the cauliflower sauce
over the top of the rice mixture and sprinkle Parmesan
cheese over the top.

Makes 6 servings
Each serving contains approximately:
1/2 fat exchange
1-1/2 vegetable exchanges
1/2 bread exchange
3/4 high-fat meat exchange
1/4 medium-fat meat exchange
187 calories

VARIATION: This is good prepared with almost any vegetable. Check the vegetable exchange list for exchange and
calorie adjustments.

Pumpkin Puff in Orange Cups

6 large oranges
3-1/2 cups mashed pumpkin
  (one 29-ounce can cooked
  pumpkin)
1 teaspoon freshly grated
  orange peel
1/4 cup fresh orange juice
2 teaspoons vanilla extract
1 teaspoon ground cinnamon
1/4 teaspoon ground nutmeg
1 egg, lightly beaten, or
  1/4 cup egg substitute
1/2 cup non-fat milk
3/4 cup seedless raisins

1. Preheat the oven to 325°F.
2. Cut the oranges in half horizontally. Remove all of the
pulp and save to use in a fruit
salad. If you have time, scallop
the top of each orange cup.

3. Put the pumpkin into a large
mixing bowl. Add both the
orange peel and the orange
juice to the pumpkin. Add the
vanilla, cinnamon and nutmeg.
4. Combine the egg with the
milk and add to the pumpkin.
Beat the pumpkin mixture with
an electric mixer or rotary hand
beater until fluffy. Fold in the
raisins and mix thoroughly.
5. Divide the pumpkin mixture
evenly into the 12 orange cups
and bake in the preheated
oven for 30 minutes. If you are
making this in advance, do not
bake it until you are ready to
serve it.

Makes 12 servings
Each serving contains approximately:
1/2 vegetable exchange
1/2 fruit exchange
33 calories

VARIATIONS:

NUTTY PUMPKIN PUFF IN ORANGE
CUPS: Omit the raisins and add
1/2 cup of chopped toasted
walnuts. Eliminate the 1/2 fruit
exchange and 20 calories and
add 1/4 fat exchange and 12
calories, for an overall reduction of 8 calories per serving.

PUMPKIN PUFF CASSEROLE: Omit
the orange cups and pour the
pumpkin mixture into an 8-cup
casserole and bake in a 325°F
oven for 30 minutes.

Garden Pasta

2 spaghetti squash
6 cups (1-1/2 quarts) Secret Spaghetti Sauce, page 48, heated
1 cup crumbled hoop (bakers') cheese or farmers' cheese (4 ounces)
1/2 cup grated Parmesan cheese
8 parsley sprigs for garnish (optional)

1. Preheat the oven to 350°F. Cut the squash in half with a heavy knife and remove and discard the seeds. (You may cut it either crosswise or lengthwise; the latter will give you longer strands.)
2. Place the halves, cut side down, in baking dishes and bake in the preheated oven for 1 hour or until fork tender.
3. Remove from the oven and, with a fork, pull the cooked flesh in strands from the skin.
4. Put 1 cup of the "spaghetti" strands on each plate. Pour 3/4 cup of the Secret Spaghetti Sauce over each serving.
5. Sprinkle 2 tablespoons of hoop cheese and 1 tablespoon of Parmesan cheese over the top of each serving. Garnish with parsley sprigs, if desired.

Makes 8 servings
Each serving contains approximately:
4 vegetable exchanges
1/4 medium-fat meat exchange
1/2 low-fat meat exchange
147 calories

VARIATION:

GREEN GARDEN PASTA: Substitute 8 cups (2 quarts) cooked green pasta for the spaghetti squash. Subtract 1 vegetable exchange and add 2 bread exchanges and 115 calories per serving.

Zucchini Lasagna

4 large zucchini, cut into 1/4-inch-thick slices
4 cups (1 quart) Secret Spaghetti Sauce, page 48
1-1/2 cups partially skimmed ricotta cheese
1 large onion, thinly sliced
2 cups grated mozzarella cheese (8 ounces)
1/2 cup grated Parmesan cheese

1. Preheat the oven to 350°F.
2. Spread half of the Secret Spaghetti Sauce in a 9- by 13-inch casserole or baking dish.
3. Top with half of the zucchini slices.
4. Add a layer of all of the ricotta cheese.
5. Spread the sliced onions on top of the ricotta cheese and sprinkle half of the grated mozzarella cheese over the top.
6. Top with the remaining zucchini and the remaining sauce, and then the remaining mozzarella cheese.
7. Sprinkle the grated Parmesan cheese evenly over the top of the entire dish.
8. Bake in the preheated oven for 1 hour or until the zucchini is tender.

Makes 8 servings
Each serving contains approximately:
3 vegetable exchanges
2 medium-fat meat exchanges
225 calories

VARIATIONS:

SUMMER SQUASH LASAGNA: Substitute 6 summer squash for the zucchini. Follow the directions exactly.

EGGPLANT LASAGNA: Substitute 1 large or 2 small eggplant for the zucchini. Slice the eggplant in 1/4-inch-thick slices. Spread in a non-metal dish, sprinkle with salt, turn slices over and sprinkle with salt again. Cover and allow to sit 1 hour. Pour the liquid off and proceed with the recipe.

Bouillon-Baked Onions

4 large Spanish onions,
 peeled and halved, or
 24 small boiling onions,
 peeled and left whole
2 cups beef stock
Dash of white pepper
1 teaspoon crushed dried
 thyme
2 bay leaves
1/4 cup minced parsley

1. Place the onions in a single layer in a baking dish just large enough to hold them.
2. Combine the stock, white pepper and thyme and mix thoroughly. Pour over the onions.
3. Add the bay leaves whole, so you can easily remove them. Sprinkle minced parsley over the top.
4. Cover tightly with a lid or aluminum foil and place in a 325°F oven for 35 minutes, then cook for 10 more minutes, uncovered, allowing the stock to reduce.
5. Remove the bay leaves and serve.

Makes 8 servings
Each serving contains approximately:
1 vegetable exchange
25 calories

VARIATION: When using large onions, make onion cups out of this recipe by removing the centers from the cooked onions and refrigerating the onion cups for future use. They can be reheated and used as little bowls for other hot vegetables or chopped meats, or served cold and filled with salad.

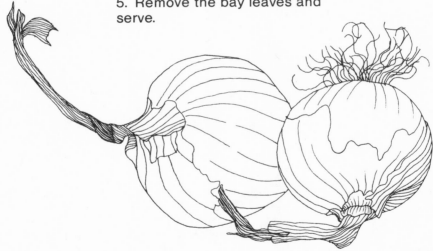

Baked Onions with Brie

4 large onions, halved
   horizontally
1 cup chicken or beef stock
4 ounces brie cheese, at room
   temperature

1. Preheat the oven to 350°F.
Place the onion halves, cut
side up, in a 12- by 7-1/2-inch
baking dish.
2. Pour the stock over the
onions. Cover tightly with a lid
or aluminum foil, and bake in
the preheated oven for 30
minutes.
3. Remove the onions from
the oven and pour off any
liquid in the dish.
4. Spread the top of each onion
with 1-1/2 teaspoons of brie.
5. Place the onions, uncovered,
back in the oven until the brie
is melted. Serve immediately.

Makes 8 servings
Each serving contains approximately:
1 vegetable exchange
1/2 high-fat meat exchange
73 calories

VARIATIONS:

BAKED ONIONS AU GRATIN: Substitute grated cheddar, Monterey Jack or crumbled blue
cheese for the brie.

HORS D'OEUVRE ONIONS WITH BRIE: Substitute boiling (pearl)
onions for the large onions
and spread each with a much
smaller amount of brie. Serve
as an hors d'oeuvre. Two whole
boiling onions with brie equal
1/2 vegetable exchange, 1/4
high-fat meat exchange and
37 calories.

Palak Paneer
(East Indian
Spinach and Cheese)

2 pounds spinach, finely
   chopped, or four 10-ounce
   packages frozen chopped
   spinach
2 teaspoons corn oil
1 teaspoon chili powder
2 teaspoons ground coriander
1 teaspoon ground turmeric
1/2 teaspoon ground ginger
3/4 teaspoon ground cumin
1/2 teaspoon salt
Dash freshly ground
   black pepper
1 pound farmers' cheese, cut
   into 1/2-inch cubes

1. Cook the spinach in a small
amount of water until just tender. Drain, reserving the liquid.
2. Put the drained cooked spinach in a blender container and
add as much of the cooking
liquid as necessary to purée
the spinach. Set aside.

3. Heat the oil in a large saucepan. Add all of the remaining
ingredients, except the spinach and cheese, and mix thoroughly.
4. Add the puréed spinach to
the saucepan and blend in
well. Add the farmers' cheese
and heat just to serving temperature. Be careful not to
overheat or the cheese will
melt.

I like this dish served with
cold sliced tomatoes, which is
the way it was served to me in
New Delhi, India, when I was
there for the Ninth International
Diabetes Federation Congress
in 1976.

Makes 8 servings
Each serving contains approximately:
1/2 vegetable exchange
1/4 fat exchange
2 low-fat meat exchanges
135 calories

VARIATIONS:
● Substitute hoop (bakers')
cheese for the farmers' cheese.
● Substitute 4 cups (2 pints)
of low-fat cottage cheese for
the farmers' cheese. Do not
add to the saucepan, but heat
to serving temperature in a
separate saucepan and put
1/2 cup on each plate. Spoon
the spinach mixture evenly over
each serving of warm cottage
cheese.

Lentil Casserole

1-1/3 cups dried lentils
1 onion, finely chopped
2 garlic cloves, minced
2 cups scraped and grated
  carrots
2 cups drained canned
  tomatoes
1/2 small green bell pepper,
  seeded and chopped
1 teaspoon salt
1/2 teaspoon freshly ground
  black pepper
1/4 teaspoon crushed dried
  marjoram
1/4 teaspoon crushed dried
  thyme

1. Place the lentils in water to cover in a saucepan and cook approximately 1 hour, or until tender; drain well.
2. Preheat the oven to 375°F. Place the lentils in a 2-quart casserole.
3. Cook the onion and garlic in a cured iron skillet until clear and tender, about 5 minutes. Add the onion and garlic and all of the remaining ingredients to the lentils in the casserole. Stir to combine thoroughly and bake, covered, in the preheated oven for 1 hour.

Makes 8 servings
Each serving contains approximately:
1 bread exchange
1 vegetable exchange
95 calories

VARIATIONS:

LENTILS AU GRATIN: Uncover the baked Lentil Casserole and sprinkle 1/2 cup grated Monterey Jack cheese over the top. Return to the oven until the cheese is melted and lightly browned. Add 1/4 high-fat meat exchange and 24 calories per serving.

LENTIL CASSEROLE WITH APPLES: Omit the carrots, tomatoes, green pepper, marjoram and thyme. Add 4 large (or 8 small) apples, unpared and diced, and 2 teaspoons curry powder with the onion and garlic. Omit the vegetable exchange and add 1 fruit exchange and 15 calories per serving.

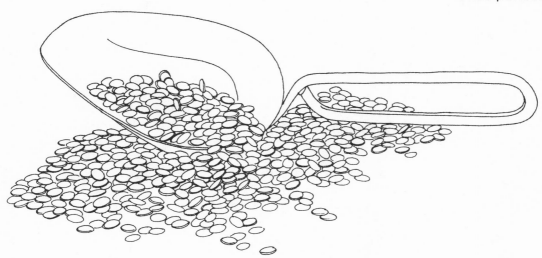

Soybean Snacks

2 cups soybeans
4 cups (1 quart) water
Corn oil for deep-frying
Salt

1. Wash the soybeans and drain them. Remove any discolored beans.
2. Put the washed soybeans in a container and pour the water over them. Cover and let soak overnight.
3. Drain the soybeans thoroughly and spread them out on paper towels to dry at room temperature.
4. Heat oil to a depth of 2 inches in a deep fryer or deep frying pan to 250°F. Add 1 cup soybeans and cook for approximately 20 minutes, or until lightly browned. Remove with a slotted spoon and place on paper towels to blot or remove excess oil. Salt lightly. Repeat with the remaining cup of soybeans.
5. Cool the soybeans completely before putting in bowls or jars. Store in a jar with a tightly fitting lid.

If you want them crisper, place the deep-fried soybeans on a baking sheet in a 350°F oven for about 10 minutes, or until they reach the desired crispness.

Makes 24 (1/4 cup) servings (6 cups)
1/4 cup serving contains
    approximately:
1 bread exchange
1/2 fat exchange
93 calories

VARIATIONS:
● Substitute seasoned salt for the regular salt.
● Substitute chili powder, cumin or curry powder for the salt for a low-sodium snack.

Mixed Vegetables and Bulgur

2 tablespoons corn oil
    margarine
1 medium onion, chopped
1 garlic clove, crushed
1 small red bell pepper,
    seeded and diced
1 small green bell pepper,
    seeded and diced
3 cups chicken stock
2 cups finely ground bulgur
    (cracked wheat)
3 cups hot cooked broccoli,
    chopped
1/4 cup chopped parsley
Lemon wedges for garnish

1. Heat the corn oil margarine in a large heavy skillet. Add the onion and garlic and sauté until tender.
2. Stir in the green and red peppers and sauté 2 to 3 minutes.
3. Add the chicken stock and heat to a boil.
4. Stir in the bulgur, reduce the heat, cover and simmer for 20 to 25 minutes, stirring often with a fork, until the bulgur is tender yet still slightly crunchy.
6. Stir in the broccoli and parsley and mix well. Serve with lemon wedges.

Makes 12 (3/4 cup) servings
Each serving contains approximately:
1/2 fat exchange
1/2 vegetable exchange
1/2 bread exchange
71 calories

VARIATION: Use any other vegetable, either in combination with the broccoli or replacing it. Check the vegetable exchange list for exchange and calorie adjustments.

VEGETABLE-BULGUR CASSEROLE: Combine the mixed vegetables and bulgur with 3 cups of chopped cooked lean meat, poultry or seafood and heat thoroughly. Serve as a main course. Add 1 low-fat meat exchange and 55 calories per serving.

Lemon Bulgur

3 cups chicken stock
1/2 teaspoon salt
1-1/2 cups bulgur (cracked wheat)
1 tablespoon freshly grated lemon rind

1. Bring the chicken stock and salt to a boil in a saucepan.
2. Add the bulgur and bring back to a boil.
3. Cover, reduce the heat to low and cook for 25 minutes.
4. Remove the lid, add the grated lemon rind, and mix thoroughly.
5. Allow the bulgur to sit for 10 minutes before serving.

Makes 8 (1/2 cup) servings
1/2 cup contains approximately:
1 bread exchange
70 calories

VARIATIONS:

LEMON-ONION BULGUR: Add 1 medium onion, finely chopped, when adding the bulgur. Increase in exchanges and calories negligible.

TUNA TREAT: Add two 13-ounce cans water-packed tuna, drained and flaked, to the Lemon Bulgur when adding the lemon rind. Add 2 low-fat meat exchanges and 110 calories per serving.

Christmas Rice Pilaf

4 teaspoons corn oil
1/2 cup minced onion
1 cup long-grain white rice
2 cups chicken stock
2 teaspoons crushed dried summer savory
1 cup diced tomatoes
1 cup French-cut green beans, cooked and kept warm

1. Preheat the oven to 350°F.
2. Heat the corn oil in a heavy iron skillet. Add the onion and rice and cook, stirring frequently, until the onion is tender and the rice is translucent, about 15 minutes.
3. Add the summer savory to the chicken stock and mix well.
4. Add the chicken stock to the rice and onions and heat until the mixture begins to boil.
5. Remove from the heat and pour the entire mixture into a casserole. Cover with a tightly fitting lid.
6. Place in the preheated oven for 25 minutes.
7. Remove from the oven and leave covered for 10 minutes before removing the lid. (You can leave the lid on much longer than this if you are waiting for another part of the meal to be ready. The rice will stay hot for a long time.)
8. Before serving, add the diced tomatoes and green beans and mix thoroughly.

Makes 8 servings
Each serving contains approximately:
1 bread exchange
1/2 vegetable exchange
1/2 fat exchange
106 calories

VARIATION:

AFTER-CHRISTMAS RICE PILAF: Add 4 cups diced cooked turkey to the rice in step 5 and mix well. Add 2 low-fat meat exchanges and 110 calories per serving. This is a marvelous way to use leftover turkey!

Mushroom Risotto

2 tablespoons plus 2 teaspoons corn oil margarine
2 tablespoons finely chopped onion
1 cup long-grain white rice
2 cups chicken stock, or as needed
2 cups mushrooms, thinly sliced (8 ounces), or one 16-ounce can mushrooms, drained
1/2 cup grated Parmesan cheese

1. Melt 2 tablespoons of the corn oil margarine in a large skillet. Add the onion and sauté until clear and tender.
2. Add the rice and cook, stirring, until the rice becomes translucent.
3. Add the chicken stock and bring to a boil. Reduce the heat to low and cook, covered, for 20 to 25 minutes or until the rice is tender. If the rice starts to dry out too quickly, add a little more chicken stock and continue to cook until the rice is tender.
4. While the rice is cooking, melt the remaining 2 teaspoons corn oil margarine in another skillet. Add the mushrooms and sauté until they are just tender.

5. Combine the sautéed mushrooms and grated Parmesan cheese with the rice. Mix thoroughly and place on low heat until the cheese is melted.

Makes 8 (1/2 cup) servings
Each serving contains approximately:
1 bread exchange
1 fat exchange
1/4 medium-fat meat exchange
134 calories

VARIATIONS:

CHICKEN-MUSHROOM RISOTTO: Add 2 cups chopped cooked chicken to the rice when adding the mushrooms and cheese. Add 1 low-fat meat exchange and 55 calories per serving.

VEGETABLE RISOTTO: Substitute 2 cups of any vegetable for the mushrooms. Check the vegetable exchange list for exchange and calorie adjustments.

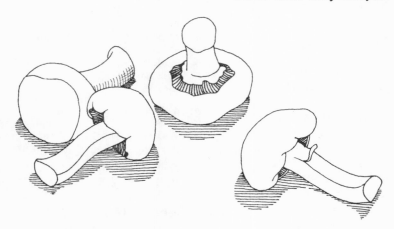

Curried Rice

2-1/2 cups water
1 cup brown rice
1 tablespoon dried minced
   onions
1 teaspoon dehydrated
   minced garlic
2 teaspoons curry powder
1/2 teaspoon freshly grated
   lemon rind
1/2 cup freeze-dried
   mushrooms
2 teaspoons powdered chicken
   stock base

1. Bring the water to a boil in
a saucepan.
2. Combine all of the remaining ingredients and mix well.
Stir the mixture into the boiling
water and bring back to a boil.
3. Reduce the heat to low,
cover and cook for 45 minutes.

Makes 6 (1/2 cup) servings
Each serving contains approximately:
1 bread exchange
70 calories

VARIATION:

CURRIED CHICKEN AND RICE: Add
1-1/2 cups chopped cooked
chicken to the cooked rice
and mix well. Add 2 low-fat
meat exchanges and 110 calories per serving.

Almond-Rice Dressing

1/2 cup chopped raw almonds
3 tablespoons corn oil
1 cup raw long-grain white
   rice
1 medium onion, thinly sliced
2 cups chicken stock
2 tablespoons soy sauce
1 teaspoon crushed dried
   thyme
1/4 teaspoon ground sage

1. Preheat the oven to 350°F.
Place the almonds on a cookie
sheet in the oven for 8 to 10
minutes or until a golden brown.
Watch them carefully, as they
burn easily. Set aside. Increase
oven heat to 400°F.
2. Heat the corn oil in a skillet
and add the rice and onion
slices. Cook, stirring frequently, until browned thoroughly.
3. Bring the chicken stock to a
boil and add the soy sauce,
thyme and sage.
4. Put the rice mixture in a
casserole dish with a tightly
fitting lid and add the hot
stock mixture. Stir and cover.

5. Place in the 400°F oven for
40 minutes. Remove from the
oven and allow to stand for 10
minutes before removing the
lid. Toss the toasted almonds
through the rice just before
serving.
   If you are making this dressing ahead of time, do not add
the almonds until after reheating,
or they will become soggy. To
reheat, add 2 or 3 tablespoons
of chicken stock to the cold
rice and mix thoroughly. Cover
and heat slowly in a 300°F
oven for about 15 minutes.

Makes 6 cups
1/2 cup contains approximately:
1-1/2 fat exchanges
1/2 bread exchange
1/4 vegetable exchange
110 calories

VARIATIONS:

WALNUT-RICE DRESSING: Use 1/2
cup of chopped walnuts instead
of almonds. Subtract 1/2 fat
exchange and 23 calories per
serving.

RAISIN-RICE DRESSING: Substitute 1/2 cup raisins for the
almonds. Add 3/4 fruit exchange and subtract 1 fat exchange, reducing calories by
14 per serving.

Herbed Brown Rice

2-1/2 cups water
1 cup brown rice
1-1/2 teaspoons crushed
    dried thyme
1-1/2 teaspoons crushed
    dried rosemary
1/2 teaspoon crushed dried
    sage
1/2 teaspoon dried grated
    lemon rind
1/8 teaspoon ground ginger
1/4 teaspoon garlic powder
1/4 teaspoon onion powder
1/8 teaspoon freshly ground
    black pepper
1/8 teaspoon cayenne pepper
2 teaspoons powdered
    chicken stock base

1. Bring the water to a boil in
a saucepan.
2. Combine all of the remaining ingredients and mix well.
Stir the mixture into the boiling water and bring back to a
boil.
3. Reduce the heat to low,
cover and cook for 45 minutes.

Makes 6 (1/2 cup) servings
Each serving contains approximately:
1 bread exchange
70 calories

VARIATIONS:

HERBED RICE-TUNA CASSEROLE:
Add one 13-ounce can water-
packed tuna, drained and flaked,
to the cooked rice and mix
well. Add 1 low-fat meat exchange and 55 calories per
serving.

COLORFUL VEGETABLE RICE: Add
1/2 cup dehydrated vegetables
(carrots, onions, celery, red and
green bell peppers, spinach,
etc.) to the ingredients in step
2 before putting into the boiling
water. Add 1 vegetable exchange and 25 calories per
serving.

Wild Rice Amandine

3/4 cup wild rice (4 ounces)
1-1/2 cups chicken stock
1-1/2 teaspoons soy sauce
1/2 teaspoon crushed dried
    thyme
1/2 cup chopped almonds
1 tablespoon corn oil
    margarine
1 medium onion, chopped
1 celery stalk without leaves,
    chopped

1. Combine the wild rice, chick-
en stock, soy sauce and thyme
in a saucepan. Bring to a boil,
reduce the heat, cover and
simmer for about 30 to 35
minutes or until all the liquid is
absorbed and the rice is fluffy.
Remove from the heat and set
aside.
2. While the rice is cooking,
preheat the oven to 350°F.
Place the almonds on a baking
sheet in the center of the
preheated oven for about 10
minutes or until a golden brown.
Watch them carefully, as they
burn easily. Set aside.
3. Melt the margarine in a
skillet and add the chopped
onion and celery. Sauté over
medium heat until the onion is
clear and tender.
4. Combine the cooked rice,
toasted almonds, cooked onion
and celery and mix well.

Makes 6 (1/2 cup) servings
Each serving contains approximately:
1 fat exchange
3/4 bread exchange
1/4 vegetable exchange
105 calories

VARIATION: Substitute 1/2 cup
chopped walnuts (15 halves,
chopped) for the almonds. Subtract 1/2 fat exchange and 23
calories per serving.

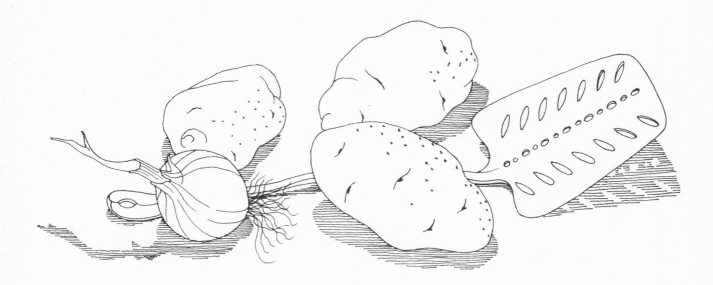

Latkes
(Potato Pancakes)

3 large potatoes, peeled and
   grated
1/4 cup grated onion
1 egg, lightly beaten, or
   1/4 cup liquid egg substitute
1/2 teaspoon salt
1/4 teaspoon baking powder
3 tablespoons matzo meal or
   all-purpose flour

1. Place the grated potatoes
in a bowl with water to cover
and let stand 12 hours.

2. Drain the potatoes well in a
strainer or colander and press
out any excess moisture.
3. Put the potatoes in a mixing bowl and add the onion
and beaten egg. Mix well.
4. Combine the salt, baking
powder and flour and slowly
add to the potato mixture. Mix
thoroughly.
5. Drop the mixture by table-
spoonfuls onto a hot, lightly
greased skillet. Cook on one
side until well browned, turn
over and brown the second
side.

Makes 16 latkes (8 servings)
Each serving contains approximately:
1 bread exchange
70 calories

VARIATIONS:

LATKES AND APPLESAUCE: Serve
1/4 cup unsweetened applesauce with each serving. Add
1/2 fruit exchange and 20
calories per serving.

SALMON LATKES: Add one 8-
ounce can salmon, drained and
flaked, just before adding the
flour mixture in step 4. Add 1
low-fat meat exchange and 55
calories per serving.

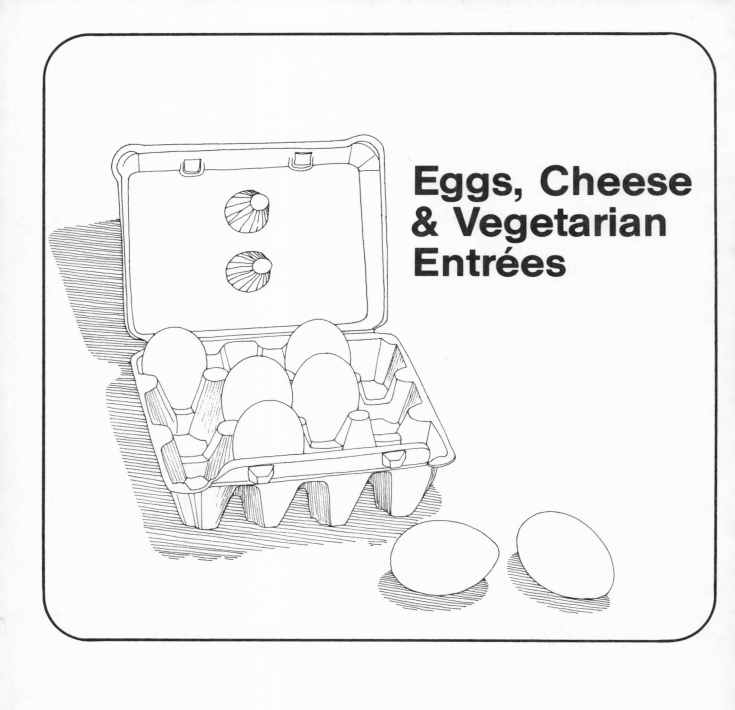

Eggs, Cheese & Vegetarian Entrées

Eggs, Cheese and Vegetarian Entrées

In most of the egg and cheese recipes in this section I have given alternate ingredients for people on low-cholesterol diets. One egg yolk contains 250 milligrams of cholesterol, and most cheeses are extremely high in cholesterol. You may wish to use egg substitute and low-cholesterol cheese in place of ingredients in recipes you are currently using. When substituting cheeses or creating new recipes of your own using cheese, check the food lists in the meat-exchange section to find out the cholesterol count per serving for specific types of cheeses. Remember, if you are allowed only 300 milligrams of cholesterol for the entire day, it is best to spread them out through the day.

Curried Easter Eggs

8 hard-cooked eggs
2 cups non-fat milk
4 teaspoons corn oil margarine
2-1/2 tablespoons all-purpose flour
1/8 teaspoon salt
Dash white pepper
1 teaspoon curry powder
1/4 teaspoon ground ginger
1/4 teaspoon Worcestershire sauce
1 teaspoon fresh lemon juice

1. Preheat the oven to 350°F.
2. Cut the eggs in half lengthwise. Remove the yolks, being careful not to tear the egg whites.
3. Arrange the egg white halves, cut sides up, in a 9-inch glass pie pan or shallow baking dish.
4. Mash the egg yolks or rub them through a sieve. Set aside.
5. Put the milk in a saucepan on low heat. In another saucepan, melt the margarine, stirring, for 3 minutes. *Do not brown.*
6. Take the margarine-flour mixture off the heat and add the simmering milk all at once, stirring constantly with a wire whisk.
7. Put the sauce back on low heat and cook slowly for 20 minutes, stirring occasionally. When the sauce has thickened, remove from the heat, add the salt, pepper, curry powder, ginger, Worcestershire sauce and lemon juice and mix well.
8. Add 1/2 cup of the sauce to the mashed egg yolks and mix well. Divide the egg yolk mixture equally among the 16 egg white halves. Pour the remaining sauce evenly over the tops of the eggs.
9. Bake in the preheated oven for 20 minutes, or until the eggs are lightly browned.

Makes 8 servings (2 halves per serving)
Each serving contains approximately:
1 medium-fat meat exchange
1/2 fat exchange
1/4 non-fat milk exchange
118 calories

VARIATION:

COLD CURRIED EASTER EGGS: After browning the eggs, cool to room temperature, cover and refrigerate until ready to serve.

Oriental-Style Deviled Eggs

4 teaspoons sesame seeds
4 hard-cooked eggs
2 teaspoons soy sauce
2 tablespoons mayonnaise
1/2 cup finely chopped
   water chestnuts
2 tablespoons finely chopped
   chives or green onion tops

1. Preheat the oven to 350°F. Place the sesame seeds on a baking sheet in the center of the preheated oven for 8 to 10 minutes, or until a golden brown. Shake the pan occasionally for even browning. Watch them carefully, as they burn easily. Set aside.
2. Cut the hard-cooked eggs in half lengthwise. Remove the yolks, being careful not to tear the egg whites.

3. Combine the egg yolks with the cooled toasted sesame seeds and all of the remaining ingredients and mix well.
4. Fill the egg-white halves with equal amounts of the mixture.

Makes 8 halves
Each half contains approximately:
1/2 medium-fat meat exchange
3/4 fat exchange
72 calories

VARIATION: Substitute Mock Mayonnaise, page 44, for the mayonnaise. Subtract 3/4 fat exchange and 34 calories per serving.

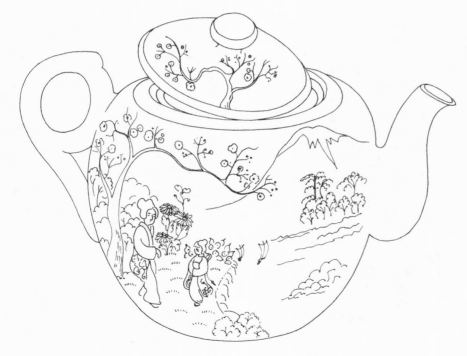

Skinny Italian Quiche

1 Perfect Pie Crust, page 166, unbaked
3 cups grated Swiss cheese (3/4 pound)
1/2 cup grated Parmesan cheese
3 eggs, beaten, or 3/4 cup liquid egg substitute
1-1/4 cups low-fat milk
1/4 cup tomato sauce
1/4 teaspoon salt
1/4 teaspoon white pepper
1/4 teaspoon ground nutmeg
1/2 teaspoon crushed dried oregano
1/4 teaspoon crushed dried basil

1. Preheat the oven to 350°F. Line a 9-inch pie pan or quiche dish with the Perfect Pie Crust dough and prick the bottom of the crust with a fork in several places.
2. Bake the crust in the preheated oven for 5 minutes. Remove and let cool. Leave the oven set at 350°F.
3. Layer the Swiss cheese and Parmesan cheese in the baked pie shell as follows: Start with 1 cup of the Swiss cheese, and top with 1/4 cup of the Parmesan cheese. Make another layer with 1 more cup of the Swiss and top with the remaining Parmesan cheese. Sprinkle the remaining cup of Swiss cheese evenly over the top.
4. Beat the eggs with the milk and tomato sauce. Add all of the spices and herbs and mix well. Pour this mixture over the cheese in the pie shell.
5. Place the quiche on a baking sheet. (This is so that if it bubbles over during baking, it will run onto the sheet rather than the bottom of the oven.) Bake the quiche in the preheated oven for 1 hour.
6. Remove from the oven and allow to cool 10 minutes before cutting to serve.
Note: If you wish to freeze the quiche, cool it to room temperature and wrap tightly in aluminum foil. To reheat, remove from the freezer 3 to 4 hours before you plan to serve it, then place in a preheated 350°F oven for about 15 minutes. This quiche makes an excellent brunch or light supper entrée. It is also good cut in small pieces and served as an hors d'oeuvre.

Makes 8 servings
Each serving contains approximately:
1-1/2 high-fat meat exchanges
1 medium-fat meat exchange
1/4 low-fat milk exchange
1-1/2 fat exchanges
3/4 bread exchange
371 calories

VARIATIONS:

BROCCOLI QUICHE: Add 1 cup chopped cooked broccoli, well drained, following the first layers of Swiss and Parmesan cheese. Additional exchange and calories negligible (about 3 calories per serving).

ITALIAN SPINACH QUICHE: Add 1 cup chopped cooked spinach, well drained, following the first layers of Swiss and Parmesan cheese. Additional exchange and calories negligible (about 3 calories per serving).

PROSCIUTTO QUICHE: Add 1/2 cup chopped lean prosciutto ham or thinly sliced cooked ham following the first layers of Swiss and Parmesan cheese. Add 1/4 low-fat meat exchange and 14 calories per serving.

Cottage Cheese Quiche

1 Perfect Pie Crust, page 166, unbaked
2 cups (1 pint) low-fat cottage cheese
3 eggs, lightly beaten, or 3/4 cup liquid egg substitute
1/2 cup low-fat milk
1/4 teaspoon salt
1/8 teaspoon freshly ground black pepper

1. Preheat the oven to 350°F. Spread the cottage cheese evenly over the unbaked pie crust (I always make the pie crust in a 9-inch quiche dish because it looks prettier).
2. Combine the eggs with the milk, salt and pepper and mix well. Pour this mixture over the cheese in the pie shell.
3. Place the quiche on a cookie sheet. (This is so that if it bubbles over during baking, it will run onto the cookie sheet rather than the bottom of the oven.) Bake in the preheated oven for 1 hour. Remove from the oven and allow to cool for 10 minutes.
   Note: To freeze and reheat, see Skinny Italian Quiche, preceding.

Makes 6 servings
Each serving contains approximately:
3/4 low-fat meat exchange
1/2 medium-fat meat exchange
1 bread exchange
2 fat exchanges
240 calories

VARIATIONS:

LOW-CALORIE QUICHE: Omit the crust and subtract 1 bread exchange and 2 fat exchanges and 160 calories per serving.

CAVIAR QUICHE: Spread 3/4 cup of sour cream evenly over the quiche. Sprinkle a 4-ounce jar of lumpfish caviar evenly over the sour cream. Add 1 fat exchange, 3/4 low-fat meat exchange and 87 calories per serving.

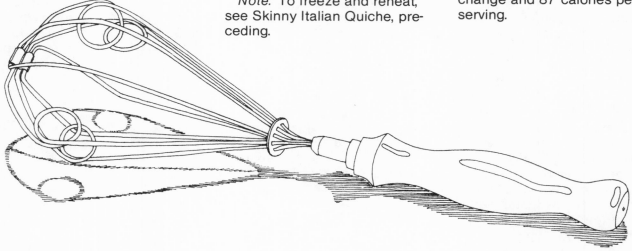

Tofu Garden Quiche
(A Low-Calorie Delight)

2 teaspoons corn oil
   margarine
1/2 medium onion, finely
   chopped
2 cups cooked chopped vegetables (a colorful assortment
   makes a prettier quiche)
2 eggs, or 1/2 cup liquid egg
   substitute
1 pound tofu (soybean curd)
1 tablespoon freshly squeezed
   lemon juice
1 teaspoon crushed dried
   oregano
1 teaspoon crushed dried basil
1/2 teaspoon crushed dried
   tarragon
1/4 teaspoon salt
1/8 teaspoon garlic powder
1/8 teaspoon ground nutmeg

1. Preheat the oven to 325°F. Melt the corn oil margarine in a large skillet. Add the onion and cook until soft, about 5 minutes.
2. Add the cooked vegetables and mix thoroughly. Remove from the heat and set aside.
3. Put the eggs and half of the tofu into a blender container and blend until smooth and creamy. Add all the remaining ingredients except the vegetable mixture and blend until smooth.
4. Pour the tofu mixture into a large mixing bowl and add the vegetables. Mix well and put into an oiled 9-inch quiche dish or pie pan.
5. Cook in the preheated oven for 50 minutes to 1 hour or until a knife inserted in the center comes out clean. Serve immediately or cool to room temperature.

Makes 8 servings
Each serving contains approximately:
1/4 fat exchange
3/4 medium-fat meat exchange
1/2 vegetable exchange
82 calories

VARIATIONS:

CHEESY TOFU PIE: Sprinkle 1/4 cup of ground Parmesan cheese evenly over the top of the pie before baking. Add 1/4 medium fat meat exchange and 19 calories per serving.

VEGETABLE TOFU PIE: Line the quiche pan or pie pan with an unbaked Perfect Pie Crust, page 166. Crimp the edges of the crust and pour in the tofu-vegetable mixture (step 4). Cook as directed in step 5. Add 3/4 bread exchange, 1-1/2 fat exchanges and 121 calories to each serving.

Cold Caviar Pie

1 teaspoon unflavored gelatin
1 tablespoon cold water
1/4 cup boiling water
2 hard-cooked eggs
1/4 cup finely chopped onion
1/4 teaspoon salt
Dash finely ground black
    pepper
3 cups Almost Ricotta Cheese,
    page 51
4 ounces caviar
Fresh watercress sprigs for
    garnish

1. Lightly oil a 9-inch pie plate and set aside.
2. Soften the gelatin in the cold water for 5 minutes. Add the boiling water and stir until the gelatin is completely dissolved. Set aside.
3. Finely chop the hard-cooked eggs and reserve 1 tablespoon for the topping. Combine the remaining chopped onion, salt, pepper and cheese and mix well. Stir in the gelatin mixture and again mix thoroughly. Pour into the pie plate.
4. Chill for several hours or overnight. Before serving, spread the caviar over the top. Sprinkle the tablespoon of reserved chopped egg on top. Garnish each serving with a watercress sprig.

This is a divinely different luncheon entrée, and, cut into small squares, it makes a fabulous hors d'oeuvre.

Makes 8 servings
Each serving contains approximately:
1-1/2 non-fat milk exchanges
1/2 low-fat meat exchange
1/4 medium-fat meat exchange
167 calories

VARIATION:

COLD CAPER PIE: Cut the cost, the cholesterol and the calories by omitting the caviar and sprinkling 1/4 cup of capers, well drained, over the top of the pie. Subtract 1/2 low-fat meat exchange and 28 calories—and the cost of the caviar.

Spinach Frittata

1 teaspoon corn oil
1 teaspoon olive oil
1 tablespoon minced onion
3 eggs, lightly beaten, or
    3/4 cup liquid egg substitute
1/4 cup grated Parmesan or
    Romano cheese
1/2 teaspoon crushed dried
    oregano
Dash freshly ground black
    pepper
1 cup chopped cooked
    spinach, well drained

1. Heat the oil in an 8-inch skillet or omelet pan.
2. Add the onion and cook until clear and tender.
3. Combine the eggs with half of the cheese, the oregano, pepper and spinach and mix well.
4. Pour the egg mixture into the skillet with the onion and cook over very low heat until the edges are lightly browned.
5. Sprinkle the remaining cheese over the top and place under a broiler until the cheese is lightly browned.
6. To serve, cut into wedges.
   This Italian-style omelet is good served hot or cold for brunch, lunch or a light dinner.

Makes 4 servings
Each serving contains approximately:
1 medium-fat meat exchange
1/4 vegetable exchange
1/2 fat exchange
105 calories

VARIATIONS:

VEGETABLE FRITTATA: Any cooked vegetables, such as green beans, asparagus, zucchini, peas or broccoli, can be used in place of the spinach. Check the vegetable exchange list for exchange and calorie adjustments.

MUSHROOM FRITTATA: Omit the spinach. Add 1 cup of thinly sliced mushrooms to the oil in the pan when you add the onions. Sauté until tender, then proceed with the recipe.

MEAT, FISH OR POULTRY FRITTATA: Add 1 cup of chopped cooked lean meat, fish or poultry in step 3, then proceed as directed. Add 1 low-fat meat exchange and 55 calories per serving.

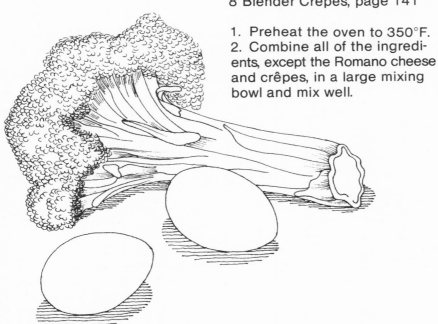

Broccoli Crêpes

2 cups partially skimmed
  ricotta cheese
4 cups chopped cooked
  broccoli
1/2 cup finely chopped green
  onion tops
1/2 teaspoon garlic powder
1/4 teaspoon salt
2 tablespoons grated Romano
  cheese
8 Blender Crêpes, page 141

1. Preheat the oven to 350°F.
2. Combine all of the ingredients, except the Romano cheese and crêpes, in a large mixing bowl and mix well.

3. Spoon an equal amount of the mixture evenly down the center of each crêpe and fold both sides of the crêpe over toward the center. Place the crêpes, seam sides down, in a glass baking dish.
4. Sprinkle the Romano cheese evenly over the tops of the crêpes.
5. Bake in a preheated 350°F oven for 20 minutes, or until the cheese is lightly browned.

Makes 8 filled crêpes
Each filled crêpe contains
  approximately:
1 medium-fat meat exchange
1/2 bread exchange
1 vegetable exchange
135 calories

VARIATION:

CREPES FLORENTINE: Substitute 4 cups chopped cooked spinach for the broccoli.

Macaroni and Cheese

3 quarts water
1 teaspoon salt
2 cups (8 ounces) uncooked
  macaroni (4 cups cooked)
2 cups grated sharp cheddar
  cheese (8 ounces)
1 cup non-fat milk
1 egg, lightly beaten, or
  1/4 cup liquid egg substitute
1/2 teaspoon salt
1/4 teaspoon freshly ground
  black pepper

1. Preheat the oven to 350°F.
2. Combine the water and salt
in a large pot and bring to a
rolling boil. Add the macaroni
to the pot, return to a boil and
cook for 8 minutes. Drain well.
3. Place half of the macaroni
in an oiled casserole and sprinkle half of the cheese over it.
Top with the remaining macaroni and then the remaining
cheese.
4. Mix together all of the remaining ingredients and pour
over the top of the macaroni.
5. Bake, uncovered, in the preheated oven for 35 to 40
minutes.

Makes 8 servings
Each serving contains approximately:
1 bread exchange
1 high-fat meat exchange
165 calories

VARIATION:

WHITE MACARONI AND CHEESE:
Substitute grated Monterey
Jack cheese for the cheddar
and add 1 cup sour cream.
When layering the macaroni
and cheese, proceed as follows: Put one third of the
macaroni in the bottom of the
oiled casserole, then top with
one third of the cheese-sour
cream mixture. Repeat layering
two more times. In step 4, add
to the egg mixture 2 tablespoons
Worcestershire sauce and 4
drops Tabasco sauce. Sprinkle
2 tablespoons of grated Parmesan cheese over the top of
the casserole. Add 1 fat exchange and 45 calories per
serving.

Peanut Butter Cheese

1 cup (1/2 pint) low-fat
  cottage cheese
1/4 cup unhomogenized
  smooth peanut butter
Non-fat milk, as needed

1. Combine the cottage cheese
and peanut butter in a blender
container and blend until smooth
and creamy. (You may need to
add a few drops of non-fat
milk to facilitate the blending.)
   This can be used as a spread
in place of regular peanut butter, and it is also delicious
spread on apples, bananas and
other fruit. It is a wonderful
way to reduce calories.

Makes 1-1/4 cups
1/4 cup contains approximately:
1 high-fat meat exchange
1 low-fat meat exchange
150 calories

VARIATIONS:
● Add enough non-fat milk to
make the mixture the consistency of sour cream and use
as a dip for fruits or vegetables.
Also use as a topping on fruit
for dessert. Calorie increase
negligible.
● Add a touch of fructose,
vanilla extract and/or cinnamon
to create a dessert. Calorie
increase negligible.
● Use on sandwiches. One
slice of bread is 1 bread exchange and 70 calories.
● Spread on muffins instead
of margarine or mayonnaise,
adding 1 bread exchange and
70 calories for each muffin
half.

Bananas au Gratin

2 cups (1 pint) low-fat
   cottage cheese
2 tablespoons fructose
1 teaspoon vanilla extract
1 teaspoon freshly grated
   lemon rind
1 teaspoon fresh lemon juice
4 bananas
4 graham cracker squares,
   crumbled
Ground cinnamon for garnish

1. Combine all of the ingredients, except the bananas, graham cracker crumbs and cinnamon, in a blender container and blend until smooth.
2. Spread the blended mixture in a shallow 7- by 12-inch glass baking dish or put 1/4 cup of the cheese into each of 8 individual au gratin dishes.
3. Thinly slice the bananas and spread the slices evenly on top of the cheese. If using individual dishes, put half of a sliced banana on top of each serving.
4. Sprinkle the top of the dish evenly with the graham cracker crumbs and sprinkle lightly with cinnamon. If using individual dishes, sprinkle half a crumbled graham cracker on top of each serving.
5. Place under the broiler until hot and lightly browned.

This is delicious for brunch, and it also makes a delicious dessert.

Makes 8 servings
Each serving contains approximately:
1 low-fat meat exchange
3/4 fruit exchange
1/4 bread exchange
103 calories

VARIATION: Any fruit, such as apples or peaches, may be used in place of the bananas. Check the fruit exchange list for exchange and calorie adjustments.

Stuffing Soufflé

4 slices whole-wheat bread
1 cup grated Monterey Jack
   cheese (1/4 pound)
1/2 teaspoon salt
1 teaspoon crushed dried
   sage
1/2 teaspoon crushed dried
   thyme
1/8 teaspoon white pepper
4 eggs, lightly beaten, or
   1 cup liquid egg substitute
2 cups non-fat milk
1/4 cup minced onion

1. Allow the bread to sit out on a counter exposed to the air for several hours so that it can be easily cubed, then cut the bread into 1/4-inch cubes.
2. Arrange half of the bread cubes in a flat shallow glass baking dish. Sprinkle half of the cheese evenly over the top of the bread. Repeat the layers.
3. Combine all of the remaining ingredients and mix well. Pour this mixture over the cheese and bread in the baking dish, cover and refrigerate overnight.
4. Remove from the refrigerator 2 hours before cooking.
5. Set the baking dish in a shallow pan half filled with cold water. Place it in a cold oven, set the oven at 300°F and cook for 1 hour. Check to make sure it is not browning too much.

This is a fine substitute for traditional turkey dressing. It is also good served with cold sliced turkey.

Makes 4 servings
Each serving contains approximately:
1 bread exchange
1 medium-fat meat exchange
1 high-fat meat exchange
1/2 non-fat milk exchange
280 calories

VARIATION:

TURKEY AND STUFFING SOUFFLE: Divide 2 cups chopped cooked turkey in half and layer one half over each layer of cheese in step 2. Add 2 low-fat meat exchanges and 110 calories per serving.

Fish & Seafood

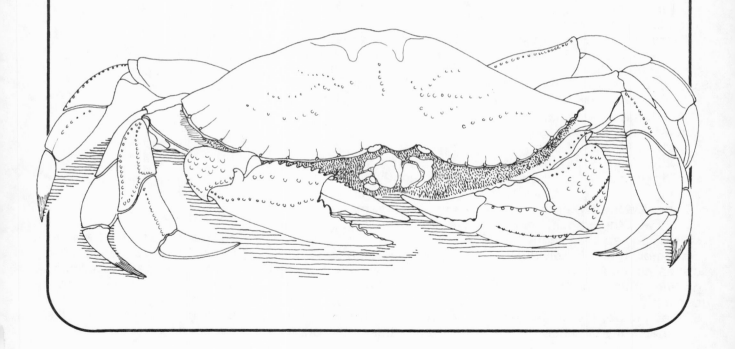

Fish and Shellfish

Fish is the best source of animal protein because it contains the least amount of fat. Most people who say they don't like fish have probably either never had fresh fish or have never had it prepared properly.

If possible, always buy fresh fish and shellfish. When it is necessary to use frozen fish, allow it to thaw completely before preparation. Prepare both fresh and thawed fish in exactly the same manner: Wash the fish in cold water and pat it dry with paper towels. Place the fish in a non-metal dish and squeeze fresh lemon juice on both sides. Cover and refrigerate it for several hours before cooking, if possible. Be very careful not to overcook the fish. You want the flesh of the fish just to go from translucent to opaque, not dried out and tasteless When sautéing, three to five minutes per side is an adequate amount of time for almost all fish and shellfish. When baking fish, it is rarely necessary to cook it more than 20 minutes before the flesh becomes opaque.

Baked Tuna in Tomato Bowls

8 large tomatoes
4 teaspoons corn oil margarine
1/2 cup finely chopped onion
1/2 cup finely chopped celery
1/2 teaspoon salt
1/4 teaspoon freshly ground black pepper
1 teaspoon crushed dried basil
Two 7-ounce cans water-packed tuna, drained and flaked
2 tablespoons grated Parmesan cheese

1. Preheat the oven to 375°F.
2. Cut a half-inch slice from the stem end of each tomato. Scoop out the pulp and discard the seeds. Chop the pulp and set it aside. Turn the tomato bowls upside down to drain.
3. Melt the margarine in a skillet. Add the onion and celery and sauté until tender.
4. Chop the reserved tomato pulp and add to the skillet. Cook for a few more minutes.
5. Remove from the heat and add the salt, pepper and basil. Then add the tuna and mix well.
6. Fill each tomato bowl with an equal amount of the tuna mixture. Sprinkle a little of the Parmesan cheese over each tomato bowl and arrange the bowls in a baking dish.
7. Bake in the preheated oven for 20 to 25 minutes or until the tomatoes are tender.

Makes 8 servings
Each serving contains approximately:
1/2 fat exchange
1 vegetable exchange
1 low-fat meat exchange
103 calories

VARIATIONS:
● Substitute 2 cups of any cooked chopped fish, lean meat or poultry for the tuna.
● Omit the tuna and add 2 cups of bread crumbs for a vegetarian tomato bowl. Subtract 1 low-fat meat exchange and add 1 bread exchange and 15 calories.

Tuna Casserole

3 carrots, scraped and sliced
3 leeks, white part only, sliced
3 cups chopped broccoli
(1/2 pound)
1-1/2 cups non-fat milk
2 tablespoons corn oil
margarine
2 tablespoons all-purpose
flour
1 teaspoon salt
1/2 teaspoon crushed dried
marjoram
1/2 teaspoon onion powder
One 7-ounce can water-packed
tuna, drained and flaked
2 teaspoons fresh lemon juice
2 tablespoons grated
Parmesan cheese

1. Preheat the oven to 350°F.
2. Steam the carrots, leeks and broccoli until they are tender but still crisp. Set aside.
3. Put the milk in a saucepan on low heat.
4. Melt the margarine in a saucepan and stir in the flour, salt, marjoram and onion powder until mixed thoroughly. Cook, stirring, about 3 minutes. *Do not brown.*
5. Gradually add the simmering milk, stirring constantly with a wire whisk, and cook until the mixture thickens, about 20 minutes.

6. Add the tuna and lemon juice and mix thoroughly.
7. Stir in the vegetables and pour into a baking dish. Sprinkle the top with the Parmesan cheese.
8. Bake, uncovered, in the preheated oven for 20 minutes. Serve immediately.

Makes 6 servings
Each serving contains approximately:
1-1/2 vegetable exchanges
3/4 low-fat meat exchange
1/4 non-fat milk exchange
1 fat exchange
145 calories

VARIATION:

SALMON CASSEROLE: Substitute an equal amount of cooked salmon for the tuna.

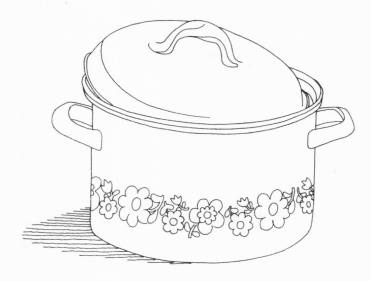

Swordfish in Caper Sauce

2 pounds swordfish steaks
Fresh lemon juice
Chili powder
1/4 cup corn oil margarine
One 3-ounce jar capers,
    drained and finely chopped

1. Wash the swordfish in cold water and pat dry.
2. Place in a non-metal baking dish and squeeze fresh lemon juice on both sides.
3. Sprinkle both sides of the fish generously with chili powder. Cover and refrigerate until ready to cook.
4. To cook, melt the margarine in a large skillet. Add the chopped capers.
5. When the pan is hot, put the swordfish in the skillet and cook about 5 minutes per side or until the flesh of the fish becomes opaque.
6. Serve immediately, spooning the caper sauce over each serving.

Makes 8 servings
Each serving contains approximately:
1-1/2 fat exchanges
3 low-fat meat exchanges
233 calories

VARIATION:

FISH IN CAPER SAUCE: Prepare any firm white-fleshed fish in this manner.

Poached Bass in Dill Sauce

One 2-pound chunk of fresh
    bass or other firm white-
    fleshed fish
1 cup finely chopped celery
1 cup finely chopped onion
1 cup coarsely chopped
    parsley
1 cup dry white wine
    (preferably Chablis)
1 cup chicken stock
1/2 teaspoon salt
Dash white pepper
1-1/2 cups Dill Sauce,
    page 44
Fresh dill or parsley sprigs
    for garnish

1. Put the fish in a large saucepan. Add the celery, onion and parsley.
2. Combine the white wine, chicken stock, salt and white pepper and mix thoroughly. Pour the wine-stock mixture over the fish and vegetables in the saucepan. If the wine-stock mixture does not completely cover the fish, add a little more wine until it does. Slowly bring to a boil.
3. Reduce the heat, cover and cook approximately 8 minutes, or until the flesh of the fish becomes opaque. Remove from the heat and allow to cool to room temperature.
4. Remove the fish from the poaching liquid and place in a shallow glass baking dish. Strain the vegetables from the poaching liquid and add them to the Dill Sauce.
5. Spoon the Dill Sauce-vegetable mixture evenly over the top of the poached fish.
6. To serve, place pieces of the sauce-covered fish on individual plates and garnish with fresh dill, if available, or parsley sprigs.

Makes 8 servings
Each serving contains approximately:
3 low-fat meat exchanges
1/4 vegetable exchange
3 fat exchanges
307 calories

VARIATIONS:
● To serve cold, after completing step 5, cover and refrigerate until ready to serve.
● Substitute salmon for the bass or other white-fleshed fish.

Steamed Salmon

6 salmon steaks, 3/4-inch thick
Juice of 1 lemon
1 lemon, sliced

1. Wash the salmon steaks in cold water and pat dry with paper towels. Sprinkle the steaks with fresh lemon juice. Cover and refrigerate until ready to cook.
2. To cook, arrange the 6 salmon steaks in a steamer basket so that they do not overlap. If steaks are too large to fit in the basket at one time, steam them 3 at a time.
3. Put the sliced lemon in the water in the bottom of the steamer and bring the water to a boil.

4. Put the steamer basket containing the salmon over the boiling water, being sure that the water is beneath the level of the steamer basket. Cover tightly and cook for 6 to 7 minutes or until the salmon is opaque all the way through. To test, pull one of the salmon steaks slightly apart in the center, using the tines of a fork. If the salmon is still bright pink and translucent in the center, it may be necessary to steam it 1 or 2 more minutes. Do not overcook or the salmon will be dry.
5. Remove the salmon from the steamer and place on individual plates or a serving platter. Serve with Dill Sauce and lemon wedges.

Makes 6 servings
Each serving contains approximately:
3 low-fat meat exchanges
165 calories

VARIATIONS:

COLD STEAMED SALMON: Bring room temperature. Cover tightly and refrigerate until ready to serve. Before refrigerating, squeeze a little fresh lemon juice over each serving.

STEAMED FISH: Steaks or chunks of any firm white-fleshed fish may be substituted for the salmon. I agree with Craig Claiborne's statement that steaming fish is infinitely superior to poaching fish in most instances. I find that it is easier to avoid overcooking by this method.

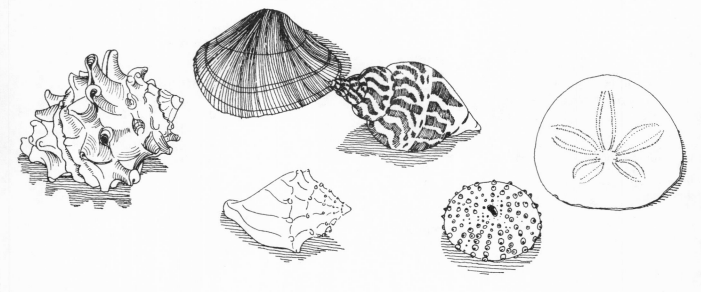

Italian Fish Dish

2 cups tomato juice
2 tablespoons red wine vinegar
1/4 teaspoon salt
1 medium onion, thinly sliced
1 teaspoon crushed dried
 oregano
1/4 teaspoon freshly ground
 black pepper
3 cups diced cooked fish
1 cup grated mozzarella
 cheese

1. Put the tomato juice in a large saucepan. Add the vinegar, salt and onion and mix thoroughly.
2. Bring the mixture to a boil, reduce the heat and simmer, uncovered, for 1 hour.
3. Add the oregano and pepper and continue to simmer slowly for another 30 minutes.
4. Combine the tomato sauce and the diced fish and mix well.
5. Spread the mixture in the bottom of a shallow baking dish. Sprinkle the mozzarella cheese over the top of the entire dish.
6. Place the dish under the broiler until the cheese is melted and lightly browned.

Makes 8 servings
Each serving contains approximately:
3/4 vegetable exchange
1-1/2 low-fat meat exchanges
1/2 medium-fat meat exchange
140 calories

VARIATIONS:

ITALIAN CHICKEN DISH: Substitute diced cooked chicken for the fish.

ITALIAN VEGETARIAN DISH: Substitute 3 cups steamed sliced zucchini for the fish. Subtract 1-1/2 low-fat meat exchanges and add 1/2 vegetable exchange for a net reduction of 70 calories per serving.

Hawaiian-Style Shrimp Curry

One 20-ounce can crushed
 pineapple packed in natural
 juice, undrained
2 teaspoons curry powder
1/2 teaspoon vanilla extract
1/2 teaspoon coconut extract
One 6-ounce can water
 chestnuts, drained and sliced
3 cups cooked shrimp

1. Preheat the oven to 325°F.
2. Combine the pineapple and juice with the curry powder and extracts and mix well.
3. Add the sliced water chestnuts and shrimp to the pineapple. Mix well and place in a casserole or shallow baking dish.
4. Bake, uncovered, in the preheated oven for 30 minutes.

Makes 6 servings
Each serving contains approximately:
2 low-fat meat exchanges
1/4 vegetable exchange
1 fruit exchange
157 calories

VARIATION:

HAWAIIAN CURRY CASSEROLE:
Add 3 cups cooked rice to the other ingredients in step 3, and then bake as directed. Add 1 bread exchange and 70 calories per serving. I like to serve the curry over 1/2 cup of cooked rice, but it's easier to serve if mixed together, especially at a potluck affair.

Fettuccine
alla Moda della Jones

3 quarts water
Salt
3/4 pound dry fettuccine
   noodles (7 cups cooked)
2 tablespoons plus 2 tea-
   spoons corn oil margarine
1 leek, white part only,
   finely chopped
1/3 cup dry white wine
   (preferably Chablis)
1/2 cup chicken stock
1/2 teaspoon salt
1/8 teaspoon cayenne pepper
1-1/2 cups low-fat milk,
   scalded
1 teaspoon fresh lemon juice
1 pound cooked shrimp
1/2 cup grated Parmesan
   cheese

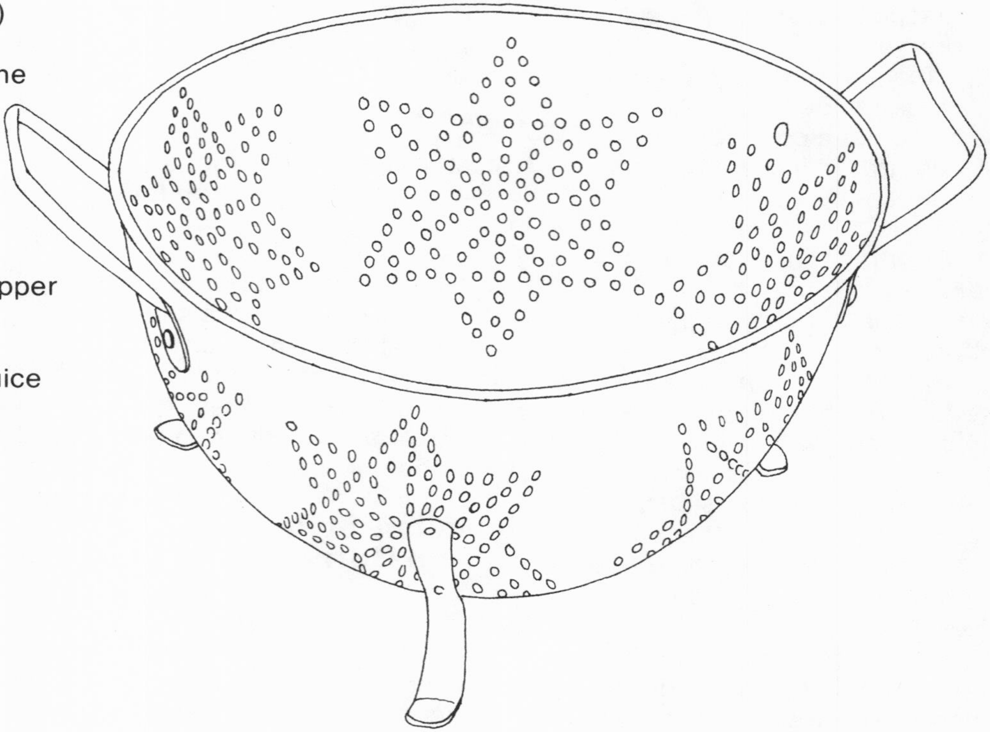

1. Put the water in a large pot, add some salt and bring to a boil.
2. Cook the noodles in the boiling salted water for 8 minutes. Drain, rinse with hot water and again drain thoroughly. Stir in 2 teaspoons of the margarine and set aside.
3. Preheat the oven to 400°F.
4. Melt 2 tablespoons of the margarine in a large skillet. Add the chopped leek, white wine, chicken stock and 1/2 teaspoon salt and bring to a boil. Reduce the heat and simmer, uncovered, until reduced by one half.
5. Add the cayenne pepper and the milk, a little at a time, and continue to simmer until the sauce is smooth, slightly thickened and reduced by one fourth.
6. Remove from the heat and add the lemon juice and shrimp and mix well.
7. Using a 2-quart casserole, put half of the noodles in the bottom. Spoon half of the sauce over the top. Put the remaining noodles on the top and spoon the remaining sauce over the top.
8. Bake 10 to 15 minutes in the preheated oven.
9. Sprinkle the top of each serving with 1/2 tablespoon of Parmesan cheese.

This may be made in advance and heated just before serving. If you are doing this, bake 25 to 30 minutes in a preheated 350°F oven, or until the sauce is bubbling. *Warning:* This recipe may become habit-forming.

Makes 8 servings
Each serving contains approximately:
1-3/4 bread exchanges
1 fat exchange
1-1/4 low-fat meat exchanges
1/4 medium-fat meat exchange
256 calories

VARIATION: Chopped chicken, turkey or any lean meat may be substituted for the shrimp.

Zucchini Marinara

6 cups shredded zucchini
2 cups shredded cooked crabmeat
1/4 cup grated Parmesan cheese
1/4 teaspoon garlic salt

1. Steam the shredded zucchini for 2 minutes.
2. Transfer the zucchini from the steamer basket to a mixing bowl.
3. Toss the crab, Parmesan cheese and garlic salt with the zucchini.

Makes 8 (3/4 cup) servings
Each serving contains approximately:
1 low-fat meat exchange
1/2 vegetable exchange
68 calories

VARIATION:

ZUCCHINI PARMIGIANA: Omit the shredded crab. Subtract 1 low-fat meat exchange and 55 calories per serving.

Poultry

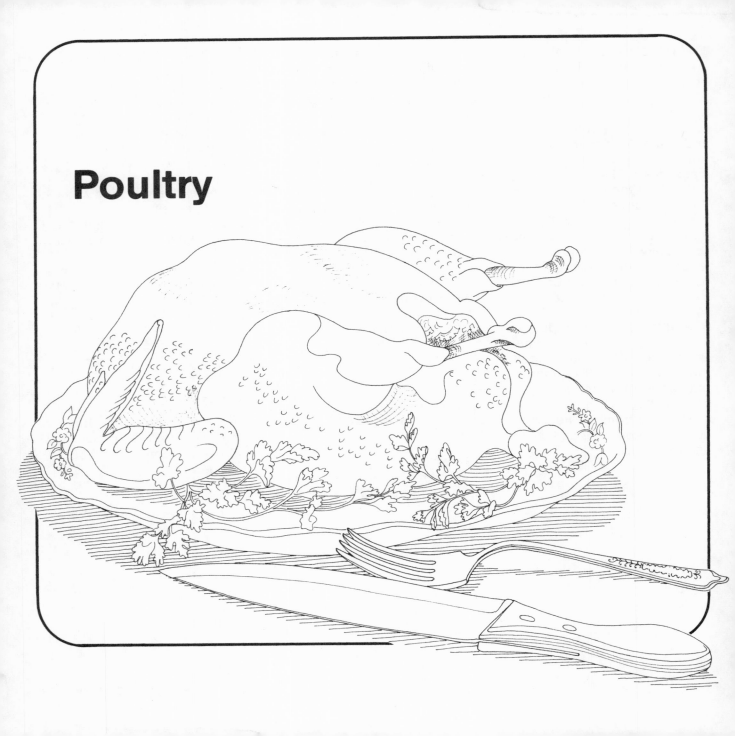

Poultry

Chicken and turkey are the best basic ingredients for recipe development. When a recipe calls for any meat, fish, shellfish or other poultry, chicken or turkey can almost always be successfully substituted. Also, from a health standpoint, chicken and the white meat of turkey, with all fat and skin removed, are two of the best sources of protein for a low-fat diet.

Roast Chicken

1 whole roasting chicken
Salt

1. Preheat the oven to 350°F.
2. Put the chicken, breast side down, in a flat roasting pan and salt it inside and out.
3. Bake in the preheated oven for about 1 hour, or until the juices run clear when the chicken is pierced with a knife.

1 slice, 3 × 2 × 1/8 inch, 1 ounce
   or 1/4 cup contains approximately:
1 low-fat meat exchange
55 calories

ROAST TURKEY: Because they are larger, turkeys roast better on a rack. If you don't have a rack, place the turkey on its side in the roasting pan and turn over on the other side halfway through the roasting. Roast at 325°F for 20 minutes per pound. If you wish to brown the breast, place the turkey on its back for the final 15 minutes.

Perfect Pâté

2 tablespoons corn oil
   margarine
1 pound chicken livers
2 tablespoons brandy
1/4 cup low-fat cottage
   cheese
1-1/2 teaspoons fresh lemon
   juice
1/4 teaspoon salt
1/4 teaspoon freshly ground
   black pepper

1. Melt the margarine in a large skillet. Add the chicken livers and sauté until lightly browned but still pink in the center.
2. Pour the brandy over the chicken livers and bring to a boil.
3. Place the livers, the juice from the pan and all of the remaining ingredients in a blender container and blend until smooth. If the mixture is too stiff to blend easily, add a tablespoon or so of water.
4. Spoon into a crock or pâté pan and chill.

I use the word "perfect" for any recipe that I feel is indeed perfect in every way—easy to make, low in calories, as delicious as I think it can be. This pâté is good served as an hors d'oeuvre on toasted rye bread, spread on toast and served with scrambled eggs for breakfast, used in a sandwich for lunch, or accompanied with cold vegetables for a summer dinner.

Makes 2 cups
1/4 cup contains approximately:
3/4 fat exchange
2 medium-fat meat exchanges
184 calories

VARIATION:

CHOPPED CHICKEN LIVERS: If you prefer the coarser texture of chopped chicken livers, blend the cottage cheese, lemon juice, salt, pepper and all of the pan juices until smooth. Chop the chicken livers to the desired consistency, using either a knife or a food processor, and combine with the blended ingredients.

Lemon Chicken— Baked to Take

3 whole chicken breasts
Salt
1 teaspoon crushed dried
   tarragon
3 lemons, halved

1. Preheat the oven to 400°F.
2. Bone, skin and halve the chicken breasts; remove all visible fat.
3. Place each halved breast on a 12-inch-square piece of aluminum foil and lightly salt both sides of the chicken.
4. Sprinkle each breast evenly with tarragon.

5. Form an envelope of the aluminum foil by first folding the foil in half, leaving the chicken breast in the center. Then fold each side of the foil over twice (about 1 inch for each fold) so that it is possible to squeeze the lemon juice into the chicken without its running out of the sides of the foil.
6. Into each envelope squeeze the juice of a half lemon. Then, holding the envelope upright, fold the top ends over twice, pressing to seal after each fold.

7. Place the 6 envelopes in a shallow baking dish and bake in the preheated oven for approximately 20 minutes.
8. Remove the dish from the oven and cool to room temperature. Refrigerate until cold.
9. Unfold the top of each envelope and pour off the excess liquid. Fold the envelope back tightly before packing for a picnic or trip.

Makes 6 servings
Each serving contains approximately:
2 low-fat meat exchanges
110 calories

VARIATION:

ORANGE CHICKEN—BAKED TO TAKE: Substitute 3 small oranges for the lemons.

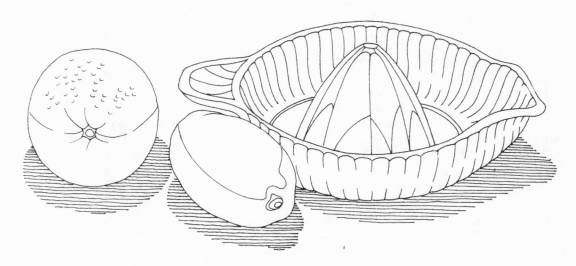

Fat-Free "Fried" Chicken
(A Bake 'n Fake)

1 tablespoon crushed dried thyme
1 tablespoon crushed dried rosemary
1 teaspoon freshly grated lemon rind
1/4 teaspoon ground ginger
1/2 teaspoon garlic powder
1/4 teaspoon onion powder
1/2 teaspoon crushed dried sage
1/4 teaspoon freshly ground black pepper
1/8 teaspoon cayenne pepper
1 teaspoon fructose
1/2 teaspoon salt
One 3-1/2-pound chicken, skinned and cut into serving pieces
Non-fat milk for coating chicken

1. Preheat the oven to 350°F.
2. Combine all of the ingredients, except the chicken and milk, in a large plastic bag and mix thoroughly.
3. Dip the chicken pieces in non-fat milk and place in the plastic bag with the mixed herbs and spices. Shake the bag until the chicken is completely coated with the mixture.
4. Bake the chicken pieces on a large sheet of aluminum foil in the preheated oven for 40 minutes, turning over at the end of 20 minutes.

Makes 6 servings
Each serving contains approximately:
2 low-fat meat exchanges
110 calories

VARIATION:

FAT-FREE "FRIED" CHICKEN, ITALIAN STYLE: Omit the thyme, rosemary, ginger, sage and cayenne from the spices, and add 1 tablespoon crushed dried oregano, 2 teaspoons crushed dried basil and 2 teaspoons crushed dried tarragon.

Enchiladas de Pollo
(Chicken Enchiladas)

1 tablespoon corn oil
1 large onion, chopped
1-1/2 teaspoons salt
2 teaspoons chili powder
1/2 teaspoon ground cumin
3 medium tomatoes, peeled and diced
2 cups chopped cooked chicken
1/2 cup chicken stock
6 corn tortillas, cut in quarters
1-1/2 cups grated sharp cheddar cheese (6 ounces)

1. Preheat the oven to 350°F.
2. Heat the oil in a skillet. Add the chopped onion and cook until clear and tender, about 5 minutes.
3. Add the salt, chili powder and cumin and mix well.
4. Add the tomatoes, chopped chicken and chicken stock to the skillet. Mix well and cook for 5 minutes over low heat.
5. In a casserole, layer the chicken mixture, tortillas and grated cheese, making as many layers as you wish, until you have used all ingredients. You should end with a cheese layer on the top.
6. Cover and bake in the preheated oven for 30 minutes.

Makes 6 servings
Each serving contains approximately:
3 low-fat meat exchanges
1 bread exchange
1/2 fat exchange
258 calories

VARIATIONS:

ENCHILADAS DE PAVO: Substitute 2 cups cooked turkey for the chicken.

ENCHILADAS DE CARNE: Substitute 2 cups cooked lean ground beef for the chicken.

Kaki's Jelled Chicken

1 whole chicken
Chicken stock
1 green onion
1 carrot, sliced
1 celery stalk
1/2 cup diced celery
1/2 cup diced carrot
2 tablespoons minced parsley
1 envelope (1 tablespoon)
    unflavored gelatin
2 tablespoons cold water
2 hard-cooked eggs, sliced

1. Put the chicken in a large
pot and add chicken stock to
cover. Add the green onion,
sliced carrot and celery stalk
to the pot and bring to a boil.
2. Reduce the heat, cover and
simmer for 30 minutes.
3. Remove the chicken from
the stock. Cool until it can be
handled and remove the skin
and bones. Cut the chicken
into pieces. Strain the chicken
stock and place in the freezer
so the fat can be removed.
4. Place the chicken pieces,
diced celery, diced carrot and
parsley in an 11- by 7-inch
shallow baking dish.
5. Soften the gelatin in the
cold water for 5 minutes. Measure 2-1/2 cups of the strained
defatted chicken stock. Bring
1 cup of the stock to a boil

and add to the gelatin, stirring
until the gelatin is completely
dissolved.
6. Combine the gelatin mixture
with the remaining chicken
stock. Mix thoroughly and pour
over the chicken and vegetables in the baking dish.
7. Arrange the egg slices over
the top of the dish, cover and
refrigerate until jelled before
serving.

   My first book was dedicated
to Kaki. She is my mother and
this is her favorite chicken
recipe.

Makes 8 servings
Each serving contains approximately:
1-1/2 low-fat meat exchanges
1/4 medium-fat meat exchange
102 calories

VARIATIONS:

JELLED TARRAGON CHICKEN: Add
1 tablespoon of crushed dried
tarragon to the stock and mix
thoroughly before pouring over
the chicken-vegetable mixture.

JELLED TURKEY: Substitute 3
cups of chopped cooked turkey for the chicken. Soften the
gelatin in a little cold turkey or
chicken stock. Bring 1 cup of
turkey or chicken stock to a
boil and dissolve the gelatin.
Proceed with the recipe.

White Chili

1 pound large dry white beans
    (2 cups)
4 cups (1 quart) water
4 cups (1 quart) chicken stock
2 onions, chopped
3 garlic cloves, chopped
1 tablespoon corn oil
One 4-ounce can whole green
    chili peppers, seeded and
    chopped
2 teaspoons ground cumin
1-1/2 teaspoons crushed
    dried oregano
1 teaspoon coriander
1/4 teaspoon ground cloves
1/4 teaspoon cayenne pepper
3 cups chopped cooked
    chicken or turkey breast

1. Combine the beans, water,
chicken stock, salt, half of the
onions and the garlic in a
large kettle and bring to a boil.
Reduce the heat, cover and
simmer for 2 hours or until the
beans are very tender, adding
more chicken stock as needed.
2. Heat the corn oil in a skillet.
Add the remaining chopped
onion and cook until tender
and clear, about 5 minutes.
Add the chopped chilies and
the spices to the skillet and
mix thoroughly.
3. Add the skillet mixture to
the bean mixture, then add the

chopped chicken or turkey breast and mix well. Continue to cook for an additional 30 minutes, stirring occasionally.

Makes 12 (3/4-cup) servings (9 cups)
Each serving contains approximately:
1/4 vegetable exchange
1 bread exchange
1 low-fat meat exchange
1/4 fat exchange
144 calories

VARIATIONS:

CHRISTMAS CHILI: Substitute chopped cooked white turkey meat for the chicken. Add 1 green bell pepper and 1 red bell pepper, seeded and chopped (or one 4-ounce jar pimientos, drained and diced, if red pepper is not available) with the chili peppers. Christmas Chili is, of course, white, red and green!

VEGETARIAN WHITE CHILI: Omit the chicken and add 3 cups of cauliflowerets in step 2 and cook until tender but still crisp.

When added to the bean mixture, further cooking is unnecessary. Subtract 1 low-fat meat exchange and 55 calories per serving.

WHITE CHILI AU GRATIN: Put each 3/4-cup serving in an au gratin dish and sprinkle 1/4 cup of grated Monterey Jack cheese over the top of each. Place under the broiler to melt the cheese before serving. Add 1 high-fat meat exchange and 95 calories per serving.

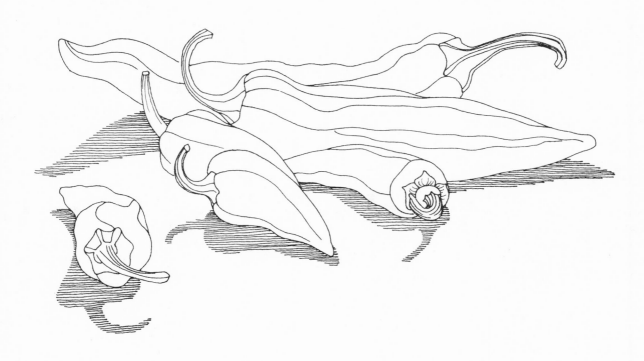

Teriyaki Chicken

1 cup soy sauce
1 tablespoon fructose
2 garlic cloves, crushed
1-1/2 teaspoons grated fresh
  ginger root, or 1/4 teaspoon
  ground ginger
4 whole chicken breasts,
  boned, skinned and halved
1 tablespoon corn oil
4 medium onions, thinly sliced
Two 16-ounce cans pineapple
  slices packed in natural
  juice, undrained (16 slices)
1 tablespoon cornstarch

1. The day before you plan to
serve this dish, combine the
soy sauce, fructose, garlic and
ginger and mix well. Let stand
overnight.
2. Marinate the chicken breasts
in the marinade for at least 2
hours before cooking.
3. Preheat the oven to 350°F.
4. Heat the corn oil in a large
skillet. Add the onions and
sauté until tender and lightly
browned, about 5 mintues. Set
aside.
5. Pour the juice from the pineapple into a saucepan and set
the pineapple slices aside.

6. Add 3 tablespoons of the
marinade to the pineapple juice
in the saucepan.
7. Add the cornstarch to the
pan and mix thoroughly until
the cornstarch is dissolved.
8. Bring the pineapple juice
mixture to a boil and simmer,
stirring constantly, until slightly
thickened.
9. Spoon half of the onions
into a shallow baking dish.
Remove the chicken breasts
from the marinade and arrange
them on top of the onions. Do
not overlap the pieces.
10. Spoon the remaining onions
evenly over the top of the
chicken.
11. Arrange the pineapple slices
evenly over the top of the
onions. Cover tightly with a lid
or aluminum foil and bake in
the preheated oven for 25
minutes.
12. Remove from the oven and
pour the pineapple sauce evenly over the top. Serve each
chicken breast half with 2 pineapple rings on top.

Makes 8 servings
Each serving contains approximately:
2 low-fat meat exchanges
1 fruit exchange
1 vegetable exchange
1/2 fat exchange
198 calories

VARIATION:

TERIYAKI LIVER: Substitute 2
pounds of calves' liver (8 slices)
for the chicken breasts. Subtract the 2 low-fat meat exchanges. Add 3 medium-fat
meat exchanges and 115 calories per serving.

Turkey Stroganoff

2 tablespoons corn oil
  margarine
2 cups sliced mushrooms
1 medium onion, thinly sliced
3 tablespoons flour
2-1/2 cups chicken or turkey
  stock
1 tablespoon tomato paste
1/2 teaspoon paprika
1/2 teaspoon crushed dried
  basil
1/4 teaspoon ground nutmeg
3 tablespoons sherry
4 cups julienne-cut cooked
  turkey
3/4 cup sour cream

1. Melt 1 tablespoon of the
margarine in a large skillet.
Add the sliced mushrooms and
onion and cook until tender,
about 5 minutes.

2. Remove the mushrooms and onions to a bowl. Do not wash the skillet.
3. Melt the remaining tablespoon of margarine in the same skillet. Add the flour and cook, stirring, until the flour is lightly browned, about 3 minutes.
4. In a saucepan, bring the stock to a boil and add it to the flour mixture, stirring constantly to form a smooth sauce.
5. Add the tomato paste, paprika, basil, nutmeg and sherry and simmer for 10 minutes.
6. Add the turkey, mushrooms and onions to the pan and simmer for 10 minutes.
7. Add the sour cream and mix thoroughly.
8. Serve immediately over whole-wheat noodles.

Makes 8 servings
Each serving (without noodles) contains approximately:
2 low-fat meat exchanges
1-1/2 fat exchanges
178 calories

VARIATIONS:

CHICKEN STROGANOFF: Substitute 4 cups julienne-cut cooked chicken for the turkey.

BEEF STROGANOFF: Substitute 4 cups cooked lean ground beef for the turkey.

Cornish Game Hens á l'Orange

4 Cornish game hens, halved
1 teaspoon salt
1 teaspoon freshly ground black pepper
2 large onions, quartered
One 6-ounce can unsweetened frozen orange juice concentrate, thawed
2 cups chicken stock
1 teaspoon crushed dried thyme
1 large orange, unpeeled and thinly sliced, for garnish
Parsley sprigs for garnish

1. Preheat the oven to 350°F.
2. Sprinkle both sides of each game hen half with salt and pepper.
3. Place each game hen half, cut side down, on top of an onion quarter in a shallow baking dish and place in the preheated oven for 15 minutes.
4. Combine the orange juice concentrate, chicken stock and thyme and mix thoroughly.

5. Remove the game hens from the oven and pour the orange-juice mixture over them.
6. Place the game hens back in the oven and cook for 45 more minutes, basting frequently. When the game hens are done, keep them warm until ready to serve.
7. Pour all of the cooking liquid from the baking dish into a bowl and put it into the freezer. When the fat has solidified on the top (about 30 minutes), remove and discard the fat and reheat the sauce.
8. Place the game hens on a serving platter, cut side down, and garnish with the orange slices and parsley sprigs. Serve with the sauce.

Makes 8 servings
Each serving contains approximately:
2 low-fat exchanges
1/4 fruit exchange
120 calories

VARIATION:

SHERRIED CORNISH GAME HENS A L'ORANGE: Substitute 2 cups of sherry for the chicken stock and 1 teaspoon of ground ginger for the thyme. Garnish each plate with an orange slice and a large parsley sprig. Serve with Wild Rice Pilaf and a vegetable medley.

Meat

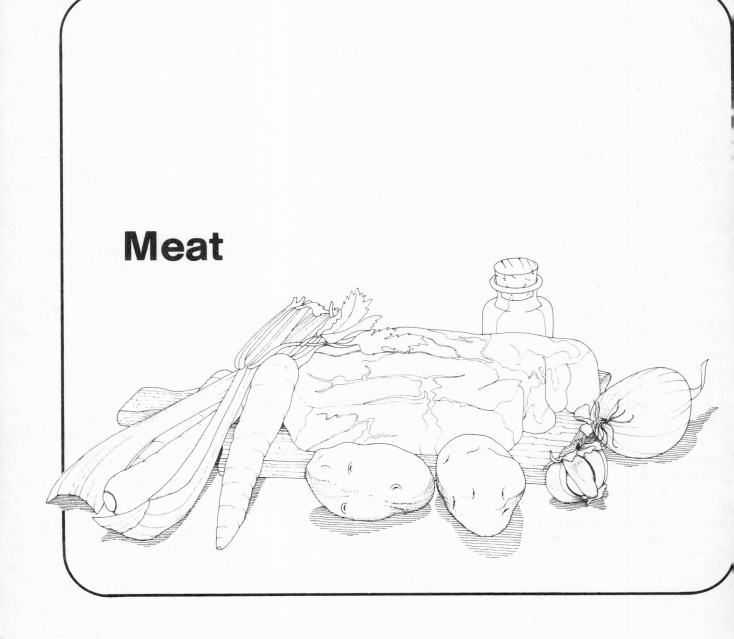

Meat

Red meat contains proportionately more fat than either fish or poultry and, in the opinion of most nutritionists, should be eaten occasionally rather than regularly. For this reason, I think that recipes for red-meat and organ-meat dishes should be truly outstanding. In this section I have tried to offer unusual preparations of inexpensive cuts.

Mustard Steak

1 tablespoon dry mustard
1/2 teaspoon salt
1/2 teaspoon freshly ground black pepper
6 cube steaks (1-1/2 pounds)
3 tablespoons corn oil margarine
3 tablespoons fresh lemon juice
1/4 cup chopped chives or green onion tops
1 tablespoon Worcestershire sauce
3 cups sliced mushrooms (3/4 pound)

1. Combine the mustard, salt and pepper and rub into the sides of each of the steaks. Set aside.
2. Melt the corn oil margarine in a skillet. Add the steaks and cook 2 minutes on each side over very high heat. Remove to a warm platter and keep warm while preparing the sauce. Do not wash the skillet.
3. Using the same skillet, add the lemon juice, chives and Worcestershire sauce to the pan juices. Lower the heat, add the mushrooms and cook until tender. Spoon the mushroom sauce over the steaks.

Makes 6 servings
Each serving contains approximately:
3 low-fat meat exchanges
1-1/2 fat exchanges
1/2 vegetable exchange
246 calories

VARIATION:

MUSTARD BURGERS: Substitute 1-1/2 pounds lean ground beef for the cube steaks. Form into 6 patties and follow the basic recipe.

Deviled Meatballs

1 pound lean ground beef
1/2 cup chili sauce
2 teaspoons prepared horseradish
1/2 cup minced onion
2 teaspoons Worcestershire sauce
1/2 teaspoon salt
2 tablespoons corn oil

1. Combine all of the ingredients except the corn oil in a mixing bowl and mix thoroughly.
2. Form the meat mixture into 24 meatballs about 1 inch in diameter.
3. Heat the corn oil in a large skillet. Brown the meatballs on all sides and reduce the heat to simmer. Cook to desired doneness.

Makes approximately 24 meatballs
Each meatball contains approximately:
1/4 fat exchange
1/2 low-fat meat exchange
1/4 vegetable exchange
47 calories

VARIATION:

DEVILED POULTRY BALLS: Substitute ground chicken or turkey breast meat for the ground beef.

Beef Jerky

2 pounds flank steak
1/2 cup soy sauce
1/4 teaspoon garlic powder
Freshly ground black
    pepper

1. Trim all visible fat from the flank steak. (Jerky keeps indefinitely if all fat is removed.)
2. Cut the flank steak lengthwise with the grain into 22 long, thin strips.
3. Combine the soy sauce and garlic powder and pour over the beef strips. Marinate for 1 hour. Remove from the marinade and sprinkle with pepper to taste.
4. Arrange the beef strips so that they do not overlap on a wire rack over a baking sheet.
5. Bake at 150° to 175°F for 10 to 12 hours. Store in an airtight container.

Makes 22 servings
Each serving contains approximately:
1 low-fat meat exchange
55 calories

VARIATION:

TERIYAKI JERKY: Omit the black pepper and add 1 tablespoon fructose and 1/4 teaspoon ground ginger to the marinade. The fructose adds about 2 calories per serving.

New England Boiled Dinner

One 3- to 4-pound fresh lean
    beef brisket
4 garlic cloves, halved
1 onion, chopped
3 bay leaves
1/2 teaspoon whole
    peppercorns
1/2 teaspoon salt
2 tablespoons pickling spices
4 medium onions, halved
8 small carrots, halved
4 potatoes, peeled and
    quartered
4 celery stalks without leaves,
    cut into pieces
2 heads cabbage, quartered

1. Put the beef brisket in a large saucepan or soup kettle and cover it with cold water. Add the garlic, onion, bay leaves, peppercorns, salt and pickling spices and bring to a boil.
2. Reduce the heat to low and simmer, covered, with the lid slightly ajar, for 3 to 4 hours (about 1 hour per pound of meat). *Stop.* Refrigerate uncovered, overnight.
3. Before reheating, remove all of the fat from the surface. Bring the brisket and stock mixture slowly to a boil. Add the onions, carrots, potatoes and celery and cook for 30 minutes.
4. Add the cabbage and cook for approximately 15 to 20 more minutes, or until the cabbage can be pierced easily with a fork. Do not overcook the cabbage or it will become mushy.
    Serve with Raisin Mustard Sauce.

Makes 8 servings
Each serving contains approximately:
1 medium-fat meat exchange for
    each 2×3×1/8-inch slice of meat
    of meat
1 bread exchange
1 vegetable exchange
170 calories (add 75 calories for each
    additional medium-fat meat
    exchange)

VARIATIONS:

CORNED BEEF DINNER: Substitute a 3- to 4-pound corned beef brisket for the fresh beef brisket.

BOILED TONGUE DINNER: Substitute a 3-pound fresh beef tongue for the beef brisket. See step 3 of Tongue in Raisin Sauce, page 127, for preparation of the tongue after it is cooked.

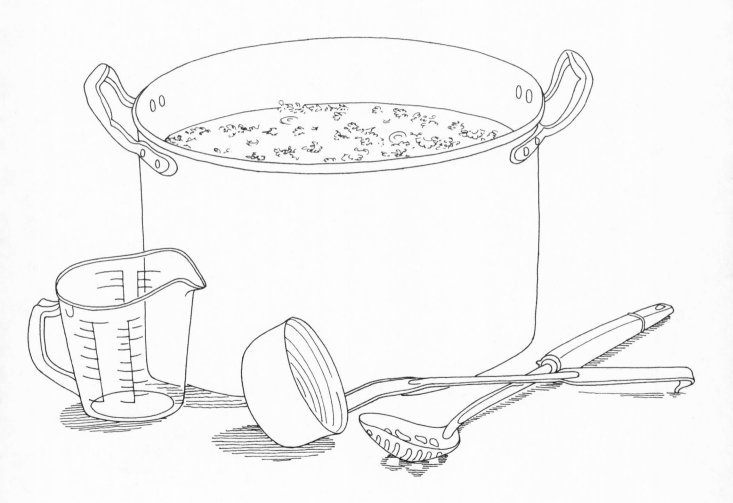

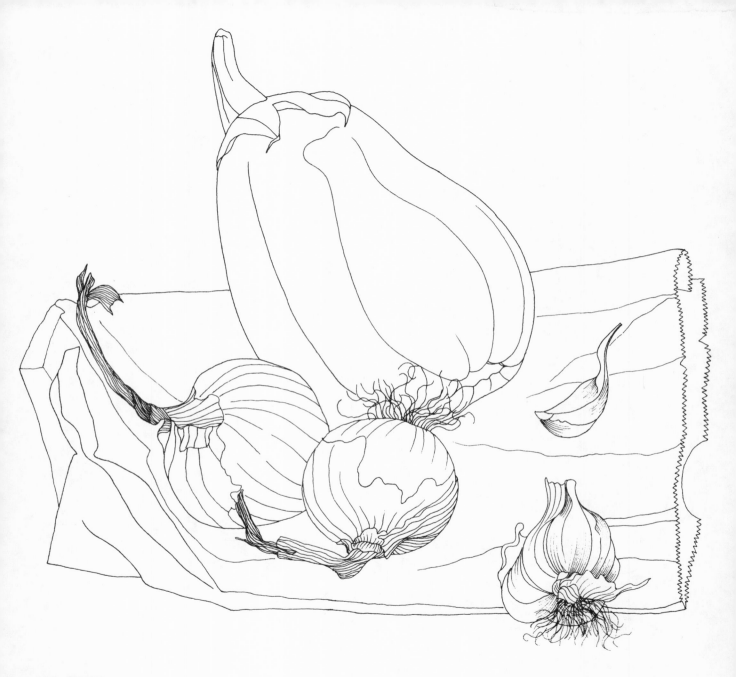

Moussaka

3 small or 2 large eggplants
Salt
2 teaspoons corn oil
2 teaspoons olive oil
2 onions, minced
2 garlic cloves, finely chopped
1-1/2 pounds lean ground
  lamb (3 cups)
1/4 cup finely chopped
  parsley
One 8-ounce can tomato
  sauce
1/2 cup dry red wine
1/4 teaspoon ground mace
1 teaspoon crushed dried
  oregano
1/2 cup grated Monterey Jack
  cheese
1/2 cup grated Parmesan
  cheese
3 cups Basic White Sauce,
  page 43

1. Peel the eggplant and cut it lengthwise into 1/2-inch-thick slices. Place the slices in a baking dish and sprinkle both sides of each slice with salt. Set aside for at least 1 hour.

2. Heat the corn oil and olive oil in a large skillet. Add the onion and garlic and cook until clear and tender, about 5 minutes.
3. Add the ground lamb and sauté until the meat is cooked.
4. Add the parsley, tomato sauce, wine, mace and oregano, mix thoroughly and simmer for 30 minutes, stirring occasionally.
5. Pour off all of the liquid from the eggplant and steam the eggplant until it is just fork tender, about 3 minutes.
6. Preheat the oven to 350°F.
7. To assemble the moussaka, place half of the cooked eggplant in the bottom of a greased 9- by 13-inch baking dish. Spread the meat mixture evenly over the top of the eggplant. Sprinkle half of the Jack cheese and half of the Parmesan cheese over the top of the meat. Place the remaining eggplant over the top of the cheese and pour the white sauce over the top of the entire dish. Sprinkle the remaining Jack and Parmesan cheese evenly over the top of the dish.
8. Bake, uncovered, in the preheated oven for 1 hour. Remove from the oven and allow to cool slightly before serving, then cut into 8 servings.

Moussaka is a Middle Eastern entrée with many regional variations. I like to serve it with Tabbouli Salad and Lavash, with Mediterranean Melon Balls for dessert.

Makes 8 servings
Each serving contains approximately:
1-1/2 low-fat meat exchanges
1/4 medium-fat meat exchange
1/4 high-fat meat exchange
1 vegetable exchange
1-1/4 fat exchanges
1/4 bread exchange
1/2 non-fat milk exchange
266 calories

VARIATIONS:

● Substitute lean ground beef for the ground lamb.
● Substitute 2 pounds of zucchini, sliced lengthwise and steamed, for the eggplant.

VEGETARIAN MOUSSAKA: Substitute 4 cups of shredded raw zucchini for the ground lamb and reduce the cooking time in step 4 to 15 minutes. Subtract 1-1/2 low-fat meat exchanges and 83 calories per serving.

Ham Soufflé in Pepper Pots

6 green bell peppers
1 tablespoon corn oil
  margarine
1 cup finely chopped cooked
  ham
3 tablespoons all-purpose
  flour
3/4 cup non-fat milk
1 teaspoon prepared mustard
2 egg yolks, slightly beaten
4 egg whites

1. Preheat the oven to 375°F.
2. Cut the tops off the peppers and remove the seeds and ribs. Place the peppers in a kettle of water, bring to a boil and boil for 5 minutes. Drain.

3. Melt the margarine in a saucepan. Add the ham, flour, milk and mustard and cook, stirring constantly, until thickened.
4. Remove from the heat and combine with the egg yolks.
5. Using an electric mixer, beat the egg whites until soft peaks form; fold into the ham mixture.
6. Spoon an equal amount of the ham mixture into each pepper and place the peppers in a baking dish. Bake in the preheated oven until the soufflé is lightly browned and set, 20 to 25 minutes.

Makes 6 servings
Each serving contains approximately:
1 vegetable exchange
1 low-fat meat exchange
1 fat exchange
125 calories

VARIATIONS:

TUNA SOUFFLE IN PEPPER POTS:
Substitute 1 cup of water-packed tuna, drained and flaked, for the ham.

CHICKEN SOUFFLE IN PEPPER POTS: Substitute 1 cup of diced cooked chicken breast meat for the ham.

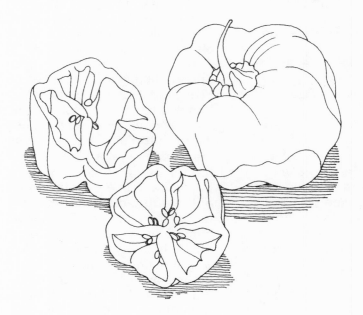

TURKEY SOUFFLE IN PEPPER POTS:
Substitute 1 cup of diced cooked turkey breast meat for the ham.

VEGETARIAN SOUFFLE IN PEPPER POTS: Substitute 1 cup of grated Monterey Jack cheese or cheddar cheese for the ham. Subtract 1 low-fat meat exchange. Add 1 high-fat meat exchange and 40 calories.

Pineapple Ham

8 slices cooked ham (1 pound)
One 20-ounce can crushed
   pineapple packed in natural
   juice, undrained
2 teaspoons cornstarch
1/2 teaspoon salt
1/2 teaspoon ground
   cinnamon
1/8 teaspoon ground cloves

1. Preheat the oven to 350°F.
2. Trim all fat from the ham and place the ham slices in a shallow baking dish.
3. Open the can of crushed pineapple and pour all of the contents into a saucepan.
4. Add the cornstarch, salt, cinnamon and cloves to the saucepan and mix well until the cornstarch is dissolved.
5. Cook over medium heat until the juice is clear and the mixture is slightly thickened.

Pour the pineapple sauce over the ham slices.
6. Bake in the preheated oven for 20 minutes.

Makes 8 servings
Each serving contains approximately:
2 low-fat meat exchanges
1 fruit exchange
150 calories

VARIATION:

PINEAPPLE CHICKEN: Substitute 4 whole chicken breasts, boned, skinned and halved, for the ham.

Chopped Ham Sandwiches

1 cup finely chopped or
   ground cooked ham
2 tablespoons mayonnaise
1 teaspoon horseradish-
   flavored mustard
1 tablespoon chopped parsley
8 slices bread
2 teaspoons corn oil margarine

1. Combine the ham, mayonnaise, horseradish-flavored mustard and parsley and mix well.
2. Spread each slice of bread lightly with 1/4 teaspoon margarine.

3. Spread 4 slices of the bread with one fourth of the ham mixture. Cover each with another slice of bread and cut each sandwich in half diagonally.

Makes 4 sandwiches
Each sandwich contains approximately:
1 low-fat meat exchange
2 fat exchanges
2 bread exchanges
285 calories

VARIATIONS:

CHICKEN SALAD SANDWICHES:
Substitute 1 cup chopped or ground cooked chicken for the ham. Substitute 1 tablespoon capers, 1/2 teaspoon salt and 1/4 teaspoon celery seed for the mustard and parsley.

● Substitute Mock Mayonnaise, page 44, for the mayonnaise. Add 1/2 low-fat meat exchange. Subtract 3/4 fat exchange and 67 calories per serving.
● Use this recipe for open-face party sandwiches and decorate them with vegetable strips, minced parsley or pimiento.
● Use the sandwich filling to make ham or chicken salad or to fill celery sticks for snacks or hors d'oeuvre.

Braised Pork with Plum Sauce

1-1/2 pounds pork tenderloin
Garlic salt
White pepper
1/4 cup port wine
One 16-ounce can water-
  packed plums, undrained
1 tablespoon cornstarch
1/2 teaspoon crushed dried
  oregano
1/8 teaspoon ground nutmeg

1. Preheat the oven to 400°F.
2. Remove all visible fat from the pork tenderloin and place the pork in a shallow baking dish. Sprinkle both sides evenly with garlic salt and white pepper.
3. Pour the port into the baking dish. Cover the dish tightly with a lid or aluminum foil and place in the preheated oven for approximately 45 minutes. At this point, check to see if the pork is done. If it is not, again cover tightly and return to the oven for 15 more minutes or until the pork is cooked.
4. When the pork is done, remove it from the liquid in the baking dish. Slice the tenderloin into round slices about 1/4 inch thick. Set aside and keep warm.

5. While the pork is cooking, make the plum sauce. Pour all of the juice from the can of plums into a saucepan, pit the plums and set the plums aside. Add the cornstarch to the juice in the pan and stir until it is thoroughly dissolved. Add the oregano and nutmeg to the pan and slowly bring to a boil. Simmer, stirring constantly with a wire whisk, until slightly thickened. Add the pitted plums to the sauce and mix well.
6. Arrange the sliced pork on a serving platter or on individual serving dishes and spoon the plum sauce evenly over the top.

Makes 6 servings
Each serving contains approximately:
3 medium-fat meat exchanges
1 fruit exchange
265 calories

VARIATION:

BRAISED PORK CHOPS: Follow the basic recipe exactly, using 6 lean center-cut pork chops in place of the pork tenderloin.

Dieter's Spicy Sausage

2 pounds lean ground pork
  (*absolutely* all fat removed
  before grinding)
2 teaspoons crushed dried
  sage
1 teaspoon freshly ground
  black pepper
1 teaspoon fructose
3/4 teaspoon garlic powder
1/2 teaspoon onion powder
1/2 teaspoon ground mace
1/4 teaspocn ground allspice
1/4 teaspoon salt
1/8 teaspoon ground cloves

1. Combine all of the ingredients in a large mixing bowl and mix thoroughly.
2. Form into 12 patties and cook in a non-stick pan until lightly browned on both sides.

  I often double this recipe and freeze the patties in individual plastic bags. The flavor improves if they are made 1 or 2 days before you plan to cook them. These patties are not only much lower in calories than any other sausage, they are even more delicious.

Makes 12 patties
Each patty contains approximately:
2 medium-fat meat exchanges
150 calories

SPICY BEEF SAUSAGE: Substitute 2 pounds lean ground beef for the ground pork. The meat exchanges become 2 low-fat exchanges and the calories are reduced to 110 per patty.

Tongue in Raisin Sauce

One 3-pound fresh beef tongue
1 teaspoon salt
1 bay leaf
1 teaspoon whole cloves
1 large onion, quartered
1 tablespoon freshly grated
   orange rind
2 cups port
1 tablespoon finely chopped
   green onions, white part only
2 cups beef stock
1 cup raisins
4 tablespoons cornstarch
1/4 cup water
1/2 teaspoon salt
Dash freshly ground
   black pepper

1. Put the tongue in a large saucepan or soup kettle with cold water to cover.
2. Add the salt and bring to a boil. Add the bay leaf, cloves, quartered onion and orange rind. Simmer, covered, until the tongue is fork tender, about 3 hours.
3. Remove the tongue from the water and allow to cool until it can be handled. Trim off all of the fat and gristle at the thick end of the tongue. Then remove the skin by slitting the underside from the thick end to the tip, using a paring knife to loosen skin around the thick end. Grasp the skin at the thick end and pull off like a glove, in a single piece. Slice the tongue, arrange on a platter, set aside and keep warm.
4. To make the sauce, combine the port and green onion in a large saucepan and bring to a boil. Continue to boil until the volume is reduced by one third. Add the beef stock and raisins and bring back to a boil. Reduce the heat to a simmer.

Mix together the cornstarch and water until the cornstarch is completely dissolved. Add the cornstarch mixture to the sauce and mix thoroughly, using a wire whisk. Add the salt and pepper and cook until the sauce has thickened slightly.
5. Pour the raisin sauce over the tongue slices.

Each slice (3 × 2 × 1/4 inch)
   contains approximately:
1 medium-fat meat exchange
75 calories
1/2 cup raisin sauce contains
   approximately:
1/4 bread exchange
1 fruit exchange
58 calories

VARIATION:

CORNED BEEF IN RAISIN SAUCE: Substitute 3 pounds of corned beef brisket for the tongue and proceed as directed.

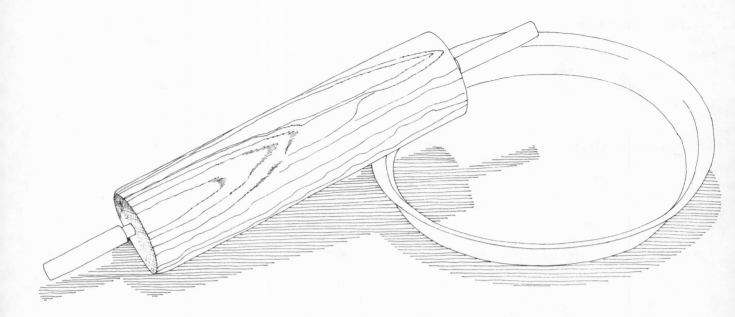

Steak and Kidney Pie

1 pound beef kidney
1 tablespoon corn oil
   margarine
1 pound round steak, all fat
   removed, cut into 1-inch
   cubes
2 cups sliced mushrooms
   (8 ounces)
1/2 cup dry white vermouth
1/4 teaspoon salt
1/4 teapoon freshly ground
   black pepper
1/2 teaspoon paprika
2 tablespoons grated
   Parmesan cheese (optional)

Crust:
2/3 cup sifted all-purpose
   flour
1/4 teaspoon salt
3 tablespoons corn oil
1 egg, beaten
1/2 teaspoon white vinegar

1. Boil the kidney in water to cover for 5 minutes. Drain, cool slightly, then remove all fat. Slice the kidney into 1/4-inch-thick slices and set aside.
2. Heat the margarine in a large skillet. Brown the kidney slices and round steak in the margarine.

3. Remove the meat from the skillet and add the mushrooms. Sauté until tender.
4. Return the meat to the skillet with the mushrooms and add the vermouth. Simmer for 10 minutes.
5. Add the salt, pepper and paprika, mix well and transfer to a deep, 10-inch pie plate or quiche dish.
6. Preheat the oven to 350°F.

7. Prepare the crust: Sift the flour and salt together. Cut in the corn oil with a pastry blender. Combine the egg and vinegar and add to the flour-oil mixture, tossing until the dough is well blended. Form into a ball and roll out on a floured board to a circle large enough to cover the top of the casserole, about 11 inches in diameter.

8. Wrap the crust loosely around the rolling pin and transfer to the top of the pie plate. Crimp the edges so that the crust is firmly in place.

9. If you are using the Parmesan cheese, sprinkle it lightly over the top of the crust. Bake in the preheated oven for about 45 minutes, or until the crust is golden brown.

Makes 8 servings
Each serving contains approximately:
1-1/2 low-fat meat exchanges
1-1/2 medium-fat meat exchanges
1-1/2 fat exchanges
1/2 bread exchange
299 calories

VARIATION:

STEAK PIE: Omit the kidney and add 1 more pound of round steak. Subtract 1-1/2 medium-fat meat exchanges and add 1-1/2 low-fat meat exchanges. Subtract 30 calories per serving.

Liver and Onions

2 pounds calves' liver
  (8 slices)
2 tablespoons corn oil
  margarine
4 medium onions, thinly sliced

1. Wash the liver and pat it dry. Set aside.
2. Melt the margarine in a large skillet. Add the sliced onions and cook slowly over low heat for at least 1 hour, or until the onions are very soft and nicely browned. Remove the onions from the skillet, set aside and keep warm. Do not wash the skillet.
3. Put the liver in the same hot pan and cook about 2 to 3 minutes per side. The liver should be slightly pink inside—overcooking makes it tough and strong-tasting.

4. To serve, spoon the onions evenly over each serving.

Many people who think they don't like liver have always had liver that has been cooked to "shoe leather" consistency. They will find that slightly pink, tender liver, smothered in onions, is delicious.

Makes 8 servings
Each serving contains approximately:
3 medium-fat meat exchanges
3/4 fat exchange
1 vegetable exchange
284 calories

VARIATIONS:

● Substitute 2 pounds of lean ground beef for the liver and form into 8 patties. Cook to desired doneness. The 3 medium-fat meat exchanges become 3 low-fat meat exchanges. Subtract 60 calories per serving.

LIVER, APPLES AND ONIONS: Add 2 large apples, pared and grated, at the time you add the onions. Add 1/2 fruit exchange and 20 calories per serving.

Northern Italian Sweetbreads

1 pair sweetbreads (2 pounds)
Pinch salt
1 tablespoon fresh lemon juice
2 tablespoons corn oil
  margarine
1 medium onion, finely chopped
1 carrot, scraped and finely
  chopped
2 tablespoons finely chopped
  parsley
3/4 cup dry white wine
  (preferably Chablis)
1/2 teaspoon salt
1/4 teaspoon white pepper
1/2 teaspoon crushed dried
  oregano
1/2 teaspoon crushed dried
  basil
1-1/2 cups Basic White Sauce,
  page 43
1/4 cup grated Parmesan
  cheese
1/4 teaspoon ground nutmeg

1. Put the sweetbreads in a bowl of lukewarm water to cover for at least 1 hour to draw out the blood. Change the water several times, if necessary.
2. Put the sweetbreads in a saucepan and add cold water to cover. Add a pinch of salt and the tablespoon of lemon juice. Bring the water to a boil, reduce the heat and simmer for 15 minutes.
3. Remove the sweetbreads and place in a bowl of cold water to cover; let stand for 15 minutes. Remove the tubes and membranes, being careful not to tear the other part of the sweetbreads. If you are not cooking them immediately, store them in the refrigerator; cover them tightly because sweetbreads tend to pick up flavors of other foods.
4. Slice the sweetbreads horizontally into approximately 1-inch-thick slices (you should have 24 pieces).
5. Preheat the oven to 350°F. Heat the margarine in a skillet. Add the sweetbreads and all of the vegetables and sauté until the vegetables are tender and the sweetbreads are lightly browned on both sides.
6. Combine the wine with the salt, white pepper, oregano and basil and pour over the sweetbread/vegetable mixture. Simmer until all of the wine is completely absorbed.
7. Remove from the heat. Combine the white sauce, Parmesan cheese and nutmeg and mix well. Add to the sweetbread mixture and mix well. Pour the entire mixture into a casserole or baking dish.
8. Place uncovered in a 350°F oven for 30 minutes.

Note: I often make this dish in the morning up to the point where it goes in the oven. Then I put it, covered, in the refrigerator and take it out at least 1 hour before baking it for dinner. I think the flavor is even better when it is made ahead of time.

This is a marvelous entrée served with vegetables and crusty Italian bread.

Makes 8 servings
Each serving contains approximately:
1/4 non-fat milk exchange
1-1/4 fat exchanges
3 medium-fat meat exchanges
1/4 vegetable exchange
309 calories

VARIATION:

FETTUCCINE WITH NORTHERN ITALIAN SWEETBREAD SAUCE: Cut the sweetbreads into much smaller pieces and serve over fettuccine noodles (or other cooked pasta of your choice). Allow 1/2 cup of cooked pasta per serving and add 1 bread exchange and 70 calories per serving.

Tripe à la Mode de Caen

3 pounds honeycomb tripe
6 slices bacon, cut into 1-inch
  pieces
2 carrots, scraped and sliced
2 onions, thinly sliced
2 tomatoes, chopped
2 celery stalks without leaves,
  sliced
1 large green bell pepper,
  seeded and finely chopped
2 garlic cloves, minced
1/4 cup finely chopped parsley
1 teaspoon crushed dried
  thyme
1 teaspoon crushed dried
  marjoram
1 teaspoon ground mace
2 large bay leaves
2 whole cloves
1 teaspoon salt
1/2 teaspoon freshly ground
  black pepper
1 cup beef stock
1 cup dry white wine
  (preferably Chablis)
Flour
Water
1 cup minced chives or green
  onion tops
1/2 cup brandy (optional)

1. Preheat the oven to 200°F.
2. Wash the tripe in at least 2
changes of cold water. Drain
thoroughly. Cut in strips about
1 inch wide and 3 inches long.
Set aside.
3. Line the bottom of a large
earthenware casserole or metal
Dutch oven with the pieces of
bacon.
4. Combine all of the vegetables
(except the chives) and the
herbs and spices and spoon
on top of the bacon. Arrange
the tripe over the vegetables.
5. Combine the beef stock and
wine and pour over the top.
6. Combine a little flour and
water to make a paste and rub
it around the top edge of the
casserole so that when you
put the lid on it creates a seal.
6. Place the casserole in the
preheated oven and cook for
at least 12 hours.
7. To serve, remove from the
oven, break the seal and remove the cover. Add the
chopped chives and brandy, if
desired, and mix well. Serve
bubbling hot.
   I like to serve this dish with
loaves of French bread and a
small, lightly dressed, green
salad.

Makes 12 servings
Each serving contains approximately:
3 low-fat meat exchanges
1/2 fat exchange
1/2 vegetable exchange
201 calories

VARIATION: For a more authen-
tic version, add 2 calves' feet
to the casserole with all other
ingredients before sealing. Add
at least 2 fat exchanges and
90 calories per serving.

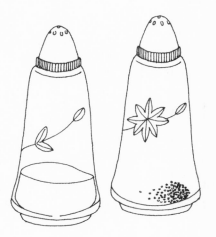

Breads

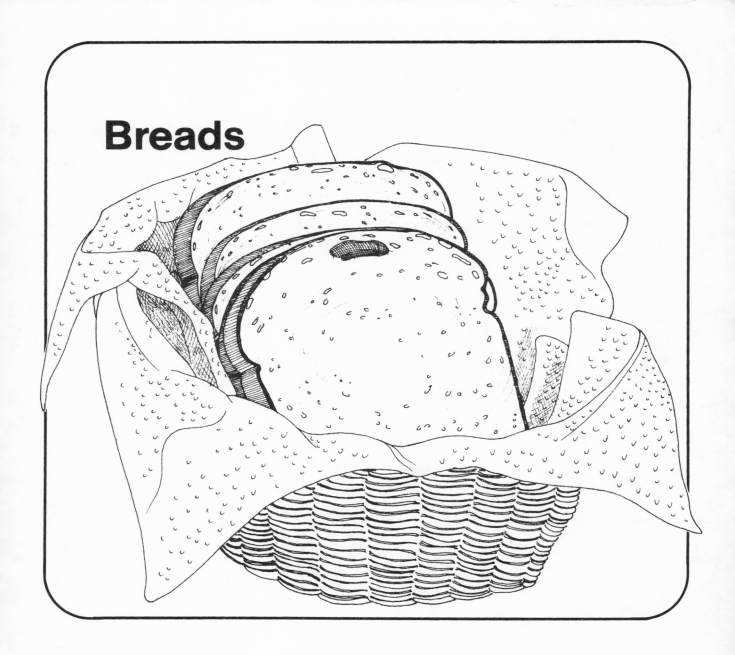

Breads

Baking your own bread can be one of the most rewarding experiences in the kitchen. Not only are fresh, homemade breads more delicious and infinitely less expensive than commercial breads, but you can also control the ingredients that go into the bread and use your imagination to create new breads.

Note: Always measure flour by dipping a measuring cup into the flour and leveling it with a knife. It is important to follow this method, because there is a surprising difference in the weight of a cup of flour measured this way and one in which the flour has been spooned into the cup, either sifted or unsifted.

Basil Bread

1 package active dry yeast (check the date on the package)
1/4 cup lukewarm water (110° to 115°F)
1 cup (1/2 pint) low-fat cottage cheese
1 tablespoon fructose
1/4 cup finely chopped parsley
1/4 cup finely chopped green onion tops
1 egg, lightly beaten, or 1/4 cup liquid egg substitute
1 tablespoon crushed dried basil
1 teaspoon salt
2 cups all-purpose flour, sifted

1. Sprinkle the yeast in the water, stir to dissolve and let stand until bubbly.
2. Warm the cottage cheese in a saucepan, transfer to a large mixing bowl and stir in the yeast mixture.
3. Add the fructose, parsley, green onion tops, egg, basil and salt and mix well. Add the flour, a little at a time, to form a workable dough. Knead until smooth.
4. Cover with a tea towel and let stand in a warm place for several hours, or until doubled in bulk.
5. Punch down the dough until again reduced to original size, form into a loaf and put it in a well-oiled, standard-sized metal loaf pan. Cover with a tea towel and let stand in a warm place until again doubled in bulk. Preheat the oven to 350°F.
6. Bake in the preheated oven for 40 minutes, or until the bread has a hollow sound when rapped with your knuckles.

This bread is delicious right from the oven. It's much easier to slice, however, when cool. Wrap cooled bread in foil and store in the refrigerator until ready to use. To serve, slice the bread and spread each slice with corn oil margarine, if desired. Reform the loaf, wrap tightly in foil and heat in a 350°F oven for 20 minutes. Or place the "buttered" slices under the broiler until lightly toasted. Remember that 1 teaspoon of margarine equals 1 fat exchange and 45 calories.

Makes 18 slices (1 loaf)
Each slice contains approximately:
1 bread exchange
70 calories

VARIATION:

ITALIAN HERB BREAD: Omit the 1 tablespoon of basil and add 1 teaspoon *each* of crushed dried basil, oregano and tarragon.

Orange Bread

1 package active dry yeast
(check the date on the
package)
1/4 cup fresh orange juice,
heated to lukewarm (110° to
115°F)
1 cup (1/2 pint) low-fat cottage
cheese
2 tablespoons fructose
1 teaspoon ground cinnamon
1 teaspoon salt
2 tablespoons freshly grated
orange rind
1 teaspoon vanilla extract
1 egg, lightly beaten, or
1/4 cup liquid egg substitute
2 cups all-purpose flour

1. Sprinkle the yeast into the
orange juice, stir to dissolve
and let stand until bubbly.
2. Warm the cottage cheese
in a saucepan, transfer to a
large mixing bowl and stir in
the yeast mixture.
3. Add all of the remaining
ingredients, except the flour,
to the cottage-cheese mixture
and mix well. Work in the flour,
a little at a time, to form a
workable dough. Knead until
smooth.
4. Form into a ball, cover with
a tea towel and let stand in a
warm place for several hours,
or until doubled in bulk.

5. Punch down the dough until
it is again reduced to its original
size, form into a loaf shape
and put in a well-oiled, standard-sized loaf pan. Cover with
a tea towel and let stand in a
warm place until again doubled
in bulk. Preheat the oven to
350°F.
6. Bake in preheated oven for
40 minutes, or until bread has
a hollow sound when rapped
with your knuckles.

This bread is delicious right
from the oven. It's much easier
to slice, however, when cool.
Wrap cooled bread in foil and
store in the refrigerator until
ready to use. To serve, slice
the bread and spread each
slice with corn oil margarine, if
desired. Reform the loaf, wrap
tightly in foil and heat in a
350°F oven for 20 minutes. Or
place the "buttered" slices
under the broiler until lightly
toasted. Remember that 1 teaspoon of margarine equals 1
fat exchange and 45 calories.

Makes 18 slices (1 loaf)
Each slice contains approximately:
1 bread exchange
70 calories

VARIATION:

LEMON BREAD: Substitute fresh
lemon juice for the orange
juice and lemon rind for the
orange rind and proceed as
directed.

Cheese Sandwich Bread

1 yeast cake or 1 package
active dry yeast (check the
date on the package)
1/4 cup lukewarm water (110°
to 115°F)
1 cup (1/2 pint)
low-fat cottage cheese
4 teaspoons fructose
1/4 cup minced onion
1 egg, lightly beaten, or
1/4 cup liquid egg substitute
1 teaspoon salt
2 cups all-purpose flour
2 cups grated cheddar cheese
(8 ounces)

1. Sprinkle the yeast in the
water, stir to dissolve and let
stand until bubbly.
2. Warm the cottage cheese
in a saucepan. Add the yeast
mixture to the warm cottage
cheese.
3. Add the fructose, minced
onion, soda, egg and salt. Mix
well.
4. Add the flour, a little at a
time, to form a workable dough.
Knead until smooth.

5. Cover with a tea towel and allow to stand in a warm place for several hours, or until doubled in bulk.

6. Punch down the dough until again reduced to original size. Place the dough on a lightly floured bread board and roll out into a long oval shape, about 1/2 inch thick.

7. Sprinkle the grated cheese evenly over the dough and roll the cheese-covered dough, jelly-roll style, to form a loaf the size of a standard-sized loaf pan.

8. Place in a lightly greased standard-sized loaf pan and allow to stand in a warm place until the dough rises just above the rim of the pan. Preheat the oven to 350°F.

9. Bake in the preheated 350°F oven for 40 minutes, or until the bread has a hollow sound when rapped with your knuckles.

Each slice of this bread is a cheese sandwich! It is delicious right from the oven. To store the bread, cool it first to room temperature and then wrap it tightly and place it in the refrigerator. I like to slice the cold bread and place it under the broiler until it is hot and lightly browned, for a toasted cheese sandwich.

Makes 10 slices (cheese "sandwiches")
Each slice contains approximately:
2 bread exchanges
1 high-fat meat exchange
235 calories

VARIATION:

MEXICAN CHEESE SANDWICH BREAD: Substitute 1 cup yellow cornmeal for 1 cup of the all-purpose flour and grated Monterey Jack cheese for the cheddar. Add 1/2 teaspoon garlic powder, 1 tablespoon chili powder and 1/2 teaspoon ground cumin in step 3. Sprinkle 1 drained 2-ounce can Ortega chili peppers over the grated cheese before rolling the dough into a loaf form.

Cornbread

1 cup white cornmeal
1 cup all-purpose flour
1 tablespoon baking powder
1/2 teaspoon salt
1 cup non-fat milk
1 egg, or 1/4 cup liquid egg
  substitute
2 tablespoons corn oil
1 tablespoon fructose

1. Preheat the oven to 400°F.
2. Combine the cornmeal, flour,
baking powder and salt in a
large mixing bowl.
3. Combine the milk, egg, corn
oil and fructose and mix well.
Add to the dry ingredients and
mix well.
4. Pour the batter into an oiled
8- by 8-inch baking dish or
pan.
5. Bake in the preheated oven
for 25 minutes, or until a golden
brown.

Makes 8 servings
Each serving contains approximately:
1-1/2 bread exchanges
1-1/4 fat exchanges
162 calories

VARIATION:

CORNY CORNBREAD: Add 1 cup
of cooked and drained corn
kernels. Add 1/2 vegetable exchange and 13 calories per
serving.

Colorful Cabbage Bread

1/2 cup finely chopped
  almonds
1/2 cup liquid fructose
6 tablespoons corn oil
1/4 cup non-fat milk
2 eggs, lightly beaten, or
  1/2 cup liquid egg substitute
1-1/2 cups all-purpose flour
2 teaspoons baking powder
1/2 teaspoon baking soda
1/2 teaspoon salt
1/8 teaspoon ground mace
1/8 teaspoon ground ginger
1 tablespoon freshly grated
  lemon rind
1 cup finely shredded red
  cabbage

1. Preheat the oven to 350°F.
Place the almonds on a baking
sheet in the preheated oven
for 8 to 10 minutes or until a
golden brown. Watch them carefully, as they burn easily. Set
aside. Leave the oven at 350°F.
2. Combine the fructose, corn
oil, milk and egg in a bowl and
mix well. Set aside.
3. In another bowl, combine
the flour, baking powder, baking
soda, salt, mace and ginger
and mix well.
4. Combine the wet ingredients
with the dry ingredients and
mix just until the dry ingredients are moistened.
5. Add the lemon rind, cabbage
and toasted almonds to the
batter and mix well.
6. Pour the batter into a well-
greased and floured standard-
sized loaf pan. Bake in the
preheated oven for 1 hour, or
until a knife inserted in the
center of the loaf comes out
clean.

Makes 20 slices (1 loaf)
Each slice contains approximately:
1-1/2 bread exchanges
1 fat exchange
150 calories

VARIATION:

LETTUCE BREAD: Substitute 1
cup of finely shredded lettuce
for the shredded red cabbage.

Bran Muffins

1 cup whole-wheat flour
1 cup unprocessed wheat bran
1 teaspoon baking soda
1/4 teaspoon salt
1 cup plain low-fat yogurt
1/2 cup raisins
1/4 cup corn oil
2 tablespoons fructose

1. Preheat the oven to 425°F. Grease 12 muffin cups.
2. Combine flour, bran, baking soda and salt in a large mixing bowl and mix thoroughly.
3. Make a well in the center of the flour mixture and all of the remaining ingredients. Mix until the ingredients are just moistened. *Do not overmix.*
4. Divide the batter evenly among the muffin cups. Bake in the preheated oven about 20 minutes, or until a wooden pick inserted in the center comes out clean.

Makes 12 muffins
Each muffin contains approximately:
3/4 bread exchange
1 fat exchange
1/2 fruit exchange
118 calories

VARIATION:

GINGER-BRAN MUFFINS: Add 2-1/2 teaspoons instant coffee powder, 1 teaspoon ground ginger, 1 teaspoon ground cinnamon and 1/2 teaspoon ground cloves to the ingredients in step 2.

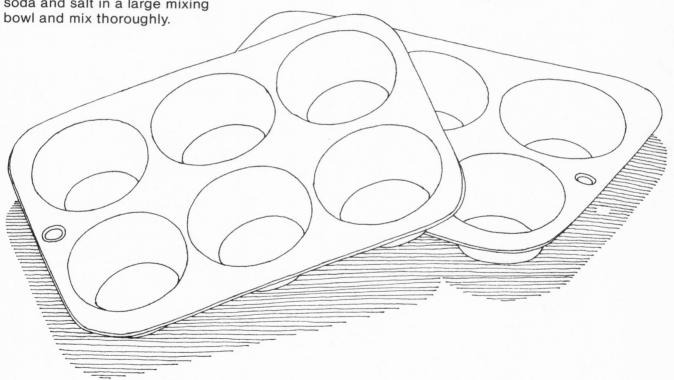

Blender Popovers

4 egg whites, at room
  temperature
1 cup non-fat milk
1 cup all-purpose flour
1/4 teaspoon salt
2 tablespoons corn oil
  margarine, melted

1. Preheat the oven to 450°F.
2. Put all ingredients in a blender container and blend at
medium speed for 15 seconds.
Do not overmix.
3. Pour the batter into 6 custard cups 3-1/2 inches in diameter or 12 muffin cups that
have been well sprayed with a
non-stick coating.
4. Bake in the preheated oven
for 20 minutes. Reduce the
heat to 350°F and bake for an
additional 20 minutes.

Makes 6 large or 12 medium
  popovers
Each large popover contains
  approximately:
1 fat exchange
1 bread exchange
115 calories

VARIATIONS:

CINNAMON POPOVERS: Add 1/2
teaspoon cinnamon to the ingredients before blending.

CHEESY POPOVERS: Pour half of
the batter into the custard
cups and cover each with 1
teaspoon of grated Parmesan
or Romano cheese (1/2 teaspoon if using muffin cups).
Add the remaining batter on
top of the cheese. This adds
1/2 medium-fat meat exchange
to the entire recipe, so it will
add 6 calories to the large
popover and 3 to the smaller
one. The result is well worth it!

Lavash

2-1/2 cups unbleached white
  flour
1 teaspoon salt
1/2 teaspoon fructose
1 package active dry yeast
  (check the date on the
  package)
2 tablespoons corn oil
  margarine, melted
2/3 cup lukewarm water (110°
  to 115°F)
Corn oil margarine for oiling
  dough
2 tablespoons sesame seeds

1. Combine the flour, salt, fructose and yeast in a large
mixing bowl.
2. Combine the melted margarine and water and mix well.
3. Slowly add the liquid mixture to the dry ingredients,
stirring constantly, until a workable dough is formed. Form
the dough into a ball.
4. Transfer the dough to a
lightly floured board and knead
until it is smooth and elastic.
Rub a little margarine lightly
over the entire surface of the
dough ball.
5. Place the dough back in
the bowl and cover the bowl
with plastic wrap or aluminum
foil. Place a hot damp towel
over the covered bowl and let
stand in a warm place until
doubled in bulk, about 1 to 2
hours.
6. Place the oven rack as low
as possible in the oven. Preheat the oven to 400°F.
7. Divide the dough into 2
balls. Evenly spread 1/2 tablespoon of the sesame seeds on
a baking sheet. Place one of
the dough balls on the baking
sheet and, with your hands,
press it into as thin a round as
possible.
8. Turn the dough round over,
spreading another 1/2 tablespoon of the sesame seeds on
the baking sheet before laying
the round down. Place the
round over the seeds and,

using a rolling pin, roll the dough out as thinly as possible without tearing it. Allow the dough to rest for 5 minutes.
9. Bake in the preheated oven until a light golden brown with darker highlights, about 15 minutes.
10. While the lavash is baking, repeat the process with the second half of dough, using a second baking sheet, and bake when the first lavash is done.
11. Cool and break each lavash into about 15 pieces.
12. Wrap crackers tightly and store in a dry place.

This Middle Eastern sesame cracker will keep for a long time if stored airtight. Some elegant restaurants serve lavash with cocktails as well as a bread to eat with meals.

Makes about 30 crackers
Each cracker contains approximately:
3/4 bread exchange
53 calories

VARIATIONS:
● Use caraway seeds or poppy seeds in place of the sesame seeds.
● Add 2 teaspoons fructose and 1 teaspoon ground cinnamon in step 1. Calorie difference per cracker is negligible.

Matzo Balls

2 eggs, lightly beaten, or
   1/2 cup liquid egg substitute
1 tablespoon corn oil
1/4 teaspoon onion powder
1/4 teaspoon salt
1/8 teaspoon white pepper
1/8 teaspoon ground nutmeg
1/2 cup matzo meal
2 to 3 quarts (8 to 12 cups)
   chicken stock

1. Combine the eggs, corn oil, onion powder, salt, white pepper and nutmeg and mix well.
2. Slowly fold the matzo meal into the liquid mixture, being careful not to overmix. Cover and allow to stand for 2 hours and no longer.
3. Moisten your fingers and form the dough into 12 walnut-sized balls.
4. Bring the chicken stock to a boil and place the matzo balls carefully into the stock. Lower the heat, cover and simmer for 30 minutes.
5. Remove the balls from the stock with a slotted spoon and serve. The balls may also be served in the stock.

Makes 12 matzo balls
2 matzo balls contain approximately:
1/2 fat exchange
1 bread exchange
93 calories

VARIATIONS:

MATZO BALLS AU GRATIN: Put the cooked matzo balls in a baking dish (or 3 matzo balls in each of 4 au gratin dishes) and pour 2 cups Mornay Sauce, page 43, over the top (or 1/2 cup over each of the 4 au gratin dishes). Bake in a preheated 350°F oven for 30 minutes, or until the sauce is lightly browned, or bake for 20 minutes and place under the broiler until the sauce is lightly browned. Makes 4 servings. Each serving contains approximately 1-1/2 bread exchanges, 1-1/2 fat exchanges, 1/2 non-fat milk exchange and 261 calories.

MATZO BALLS AU GRATIN II: Use Cheddar Cheese Sauce, page 43, in place of the Mornay Sauce, above.

MATZO MUNCHIES: Use 36 matzo crackers (the 8-calorie variety) and 2 cups of ice water. Or break large matzos (6 by 6 inches, 90 calories each) into 10 pieces each to make cracker-sized portions. Allow the matzo crackers to soak longer in the ice water before draining because of their different consistency. Six Matzo Munchies contain approximately 3/4 bread exchange, 1 fat exchange and 98 calories.

Toasted Tortilla Chips

12 corn tortillas
Salt

1. Preheat the oven to 400°F.
2. Cut each tortilla into 6 pie-shaped wedges. Spread half of the tortilla chips on a baking sheet and salt lightly.

3. Bake in the preheated oven for 10 minutes. Remove from the oven, turn each tortilla chip over and return them to the oven for 3 more minutes.
4. Remove from the baking sheet and let cool. Repeat with remaining tortilla chips.

If you prefer smaller chips, cut the tortillas into smaller pieces before toasting them. They are much fresher tasting than the tortilla chips you buy at the store and, more importantly, they are fat free.

Makes 72 chips
6 chips contain approximately:
1 bread exchange
70 calories

VARIATION: Sprinkle the tortilla chips with seasoned salt, ground cumin or chili powder.

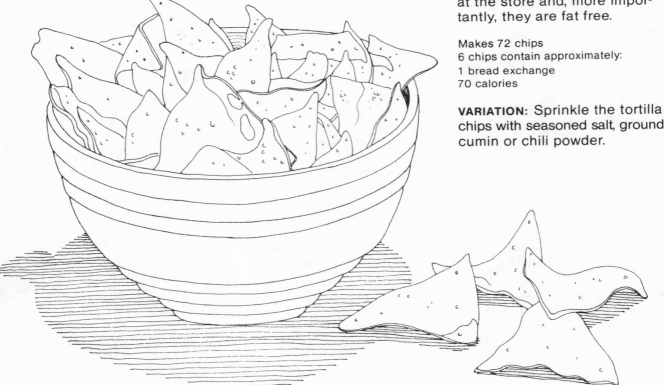

Crispier Crackers

24 soda cracker squares
1 cup ice water
2 tablespoons corn oil
  margarine, melted

1. Preheat the oven to 400°F. Arrange the crackers at least 1/2 inch apart on a well-greased baking sheet with sides.
2. Pour the ice water evenly over the crackers. When all of the crackers are completely soaked, carefully spoon the remaining ice water out of the baking sheet.
3. Brush the drained crackers with the melted margarine.
4. Bake in the preheated oven for 35 minutes or until crispy and light golden brown. Be careful that the crackers do not get too brown.

Makes 24 crackers
3 crackers contain approximately:
1 bread exchange
3/4 fat exchange
104 calories

Blender Crêpes

1 cup non-fat milk
3/4 cup all-purpose flour
1/4 teaspoon salt
2 eggs, lightly beaten, or
  1/2 cup liquid egg substitute
1 teaspoon corn oil margarine

1. Combine all ingredients, except the margarine, in a blender container and blend until thoroughly mixed.
2. Melt the margarine in an omelet or crêpe pan over medium heat. Tilt the pan to make sure the entire inner surface is coated.
3. Pour the melted margarine into the blender container with the crêpe batter and mix well.
4. Pour just enough crêpe batter into the pan to barely cover the bottom of the pan (about 2 tablespoons) and tilt the pan from side to side to spread the batter evenly.
5. Cook over medium heat until the edges start to curl, then carefully turn the crêpe with a spatula and brown the second side.

6. Repeat until all of the batter is used. To keep the crêpes pliable, put them in a covered casserole in a warm oven.

To freeze the crêpes, put a piece of aluminum foil or waxed paper between each 2 crêpes and wrap them well so that they are not exposed to the air. Before using, bring to room temperature and put them in a preheated 300°F oven for 20 minutes, or until they are soft and pliable. If you do not reheat the crêpes, they will break when you try to fold them.

Makes 15 crêpes
Each crêpe contains approximately:
1/2 bread exchange
35 calories

VARIATIONS:

CINNAMON CREPES: Add 1/2 teaspoon ground cinnamon to the batter.

CHEESY CREPES: Add 2 tablespoons grated Parmesan or Romano cheese to the batter. Calories added are negligible.

Oatmeal Pancakes

1-1/2 cups rolled oats
1/4 teaspoon salt
1/4 teaspoon baking powder
1/4 teaspoon baking soda
1 egg, lightly beaten, or
   1/4 cup liquid egg substitute
1 cup plain low-fat yogurt
1 tablespoon corn oil
   margarine

1. Put the rolled oats in a blender container or a food processor. Blend for approximately 1 minute or until the consistency of flour.
2. Combine the oat flour, salt, baking powder and baking soda in a large mixing bowl and mix well.
3. Combine all of the remaining ingredients, except the margarine, in another bowl and mix well.
4. Combine the liquid and dry ingredients and mix until the dry ingredients are just moistened.
5. Heat a cured iron skillet or Teflon pan. Add the corn oil margarine and allow it to melt as the pan heats. When the pan is hot, wipe the margarine out with a paper towel.
6. Spoon about 3 tablespoons of batter into the pan for each pancake. Cook over medium heat until bubbles form on the surface and the underside is lightly browned. Turn the pancakes over and cook on the second side until lightly browned.

Makes eight 4-inch pancakes
Each pancake contains approximately:
3/4 bread exchange
1/2 fat exchange
76 calories

VARIATIONS:

FRESH-FRUIT OATMEAL PANCAKES: Add 1 teaspoon of fructose and 1/4 teaspoon of ground cinnamon to the batter. Before turning each pancake to brown the second side, spoon approximately 1 tablespoon of chopped fresh fruit of choice on top. This adds less than 10 calories and less than 1/4 fruit exchange per pancake.

OATMEAL HAMCAKES: Add 1/2 teaspoon of dry mustard and a dash of Worcestershire sauce to the batter. Before turning each pancake to brown the second side, spoon 1 tablespoon of diced cooked lean ham on the top. Add 1/4 low-fat meat exchange and approximately 14 calories per pancake.

Banana Waffles

1 package active dry yeast (check the date on the package)
1 cup non-fat milk, heated to lukewarm (110° to 115°F)
2 eggs, beaten, or 1/2 cup liquid egg substitute
3 large ripe bananas, mashed
2 teaspoons corn oil
2 teaspoons vanilla extract
2 cups whole-wheat flour
1/4 teaspoon salt
1/2 teaspoon ground cinnamon

1. Sprinkle the yeast in the milk, stir to dissolve and let stand until bubbly.
2. Combine the eggs, bananas, oil and vanilla extract and mix well. Stir into the yeast mixture.
3. Combine the flour, salt and cinnamon and mix into the egg-yeast mixture, a little at a time, until well blended.
4. Cover the bowl with a tea towel and let stand in a warm place for about 1 hour.
5. Bake in a hot oiled or Teflon waffle iron for about 5 minutes, or until iron indicates waffle is done.

Makes six 7-inch waffles
Each 1/2 waffle contains approximately:
1 bread exchange
1/2 fruit exchange
90 calories

VARIATIONS:

● Serve with 1/4 cup low-fat cottage cheese. Add 1 low-fat meat exchange and 55 calories per waffle.

PEACHY WAFFLES: Substitute 2 large peaches, peeled and mashed, for the bananas. Subtract 1/4 fruit exchange and 10 calories per waffle.

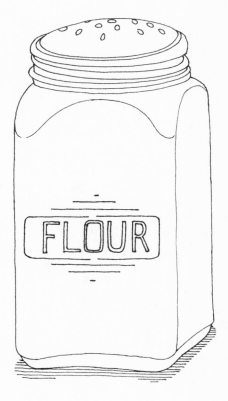

Whole-Wheat Noodles

2 cups whole-wheat flour
1-1/2 tablespoons corn oil
3/4 cup warm water
2 tablespoons salt for cooking
1 tablespoon corn oil for
   cooking

1. With a pastry blender, combine the flour and 1-1/2 tablespoons of corn oil until the mixture is well combined and is the consistency of coarse cornmeal.
2. Add the water to the flour mixture, a little at a time, until a firm ball of dough is formed. Transfer the dough to a floured board and knead until shiny, smooth and elastic.
3. Form the dough into a ball, cover with an inverted bowl and let stand at room temperature for at least 1 hour. Divide the ball of dough into 4 equal portions and wrap 3 portions in plastic wrap.

4. Place the fourth portion on a lightly floured board and flatten into a square about 1 inch thick with the palm of your hand. With a heavy rolling pin, roll out the dough into a rectangle. Turn the rectangle 180 degrees and roll it out again, this time crosswise. Continue rolling and turning until the dough is the desired thickness, about 1/8 inch or less. (To prevent the dough from sticking as you roll it out, carefully lift it and sprinkle a little more flour on the board.)
5. Cut the rolled-out dough into 1/2-inch-wide strips, then repeat with the remaining dough portions.

6. To cook the noodles, use a large (6-quart) kettle. Fill it with water and add the salt and corn oil. Bring the water to a boil and add the noodles. Boil about 8 to 10 minutes, or to taste.
7. Drain the noodles well in a colander. Serve plain, or with Turkey Stroganoff, or with your favorite sauce.

Makes 8 servings
Each serving contains approximately:
1/2 fat exchange
1 bread exchange
93 calories

VARIATIONS:

GREEN NOODLES: Use spinach flour (found in many health-food stores) in place of the whole-wheat flour.

JUST PLAIN NOODLES: Use all-purpose flour in place of the whole-wheat flour.

Peachy Pizza

2 whole-wheat English muffins
1/2 cup Peach Jam, page 148
1 cup grated mozzarella
  cheese (4 ounces)

1. Cut the English muffins in
half and roll them with a rolling
pin until each half is flatter
and larger in diameter.
2. Toast each muffin half, cut
side up, in the broiler.
3. Spread 2 tablespoons of
the Peach Jam on each toasted
muffin half.
4. Sprinkle 1/4 cup of the
grated mozzarella cheese evenly
over the top of each muffin
half.
5. Return the muffins to the
broiler until the cheese is melted
and very lightly browned. Serve
immediately.

Makes 4 servings
Each serving contains approximately:
1 bread exchange
1 medium-fat meat exchange
1/4 fruit exchange
155 calories

VARIATION: Use the Fruit Jam
variation of Peach Jam. The
fruit exchange and calories
may vary slightly, depending
upon the fruit used (check the
fruit exchange list).

Masala Dosa
(Indian Sandwich)

4 flour tortillas
1 tablespoon corn oil
1 medium onion, finely
  chopped
2 canned green chili peppers,
  seeded, drained and
  finely chopped
1 garlic clove, minced
1/4 teaspoon ground turmeric
1/4 teaspoon ground ginger
1/2 teaspoon chili powder
1/2 teaspoon ground
  coriander
1/2 teaspoon ground cumin
1/4 teaspoon salt
1/2 cup finely diced cooked
  potatoes
2 tablespoons minced parsley
1 teaspoon corn oil margarine

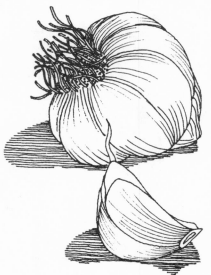

1. Preheat the oven to 300°F.
Wrap the 4 tortillas in aluminum foil and place in the
preheated oven until you are
ready to use them.
2. Heat the corn oil in a skillet.
Add the onion, chili peppers
and garlic and cook until tender.
3. Add all of the spices and
mix well. Mix in the potatoes
and parsley and set aside.
4. Remove the tortillas from
the oven and divide the potato
and onion mixture evenly over
half of each tortilla. Fold each
tortilla in half and then fold
again to form a pie-shaped
"sandwich."
5. Heat the margarine in a
large skillet. When the pan is
hot, brown each sandwich on
both sides. Cut each sandwich
in half and serve hot.

Makes 8 servings
Each serving contains approximately:
1/2 bread exchange
1/4 vegetable exchange
1/2 fat exchange
65 calories

VARIATION: Substitute 1/2 cup
finely diced cooked sweet potatoes for the regular potatoes,
for an interesting flavor variation. Exchange and calorie
changes are negligible per
serving.

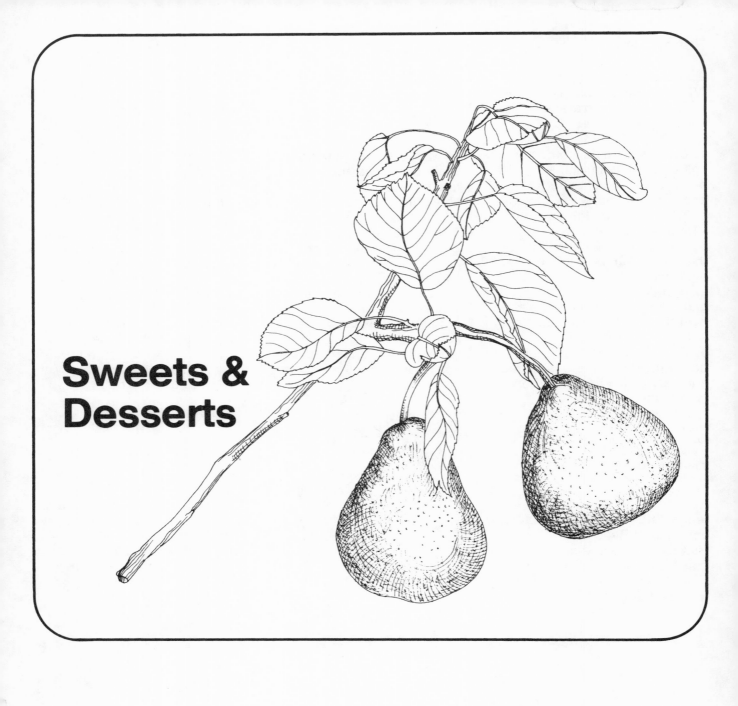

Sweets &
Desserts

Sweets and Desserts

The very best dessert for everyone is fresh fruit. Not only is it delicious, it is also a wonderful source of vitamins, minerals and fiber. When fresh fruits are not available, frozen unsweetened fruits and fruits canned in either water or their natural juices are good substitutes.

There will always be times when you want something else for dessert, however, so this section contains many light desserts based on fruits. And for those special occasions when you want a real birthday cake or a dramatic finale for a dinner party, I have included recipes for Piña Colada Cake, Cheesecake and a fabulous Lavender Soufflé.

Date "Sugar"

32 dates, pitted and sliced

1. Preheat the oven to 250°F. Spread the sliced dates evenly on an ungreased baking sheet, being careful not to overlap them.

2. Put the dates in the preheated oven for about 12 to 15 hours, or until they are completely dried out and hard. (Dates contain different amounts of moisture, so cooking time will vary.) Watch carefully so that they do not burn.
3. Turn the oven off, leave the door ajar and cool the dates to room temperature.
4. Put a few of the hard dates (and they will be *very* hard—like rocks!) in a blender container. Turn the blender on and grind them until they have all been reduced to a powdery, sugarlike substance. Continue adding dates, a few at a time, until all are the consistency of sugar.

It is far easier to buy date "sugar" at your natural foods stores, but if you can't find it, or just want to know how it is made, I have included this method. I like to use date "sugar" for sweetening in some recipes because it provides an interesting flavor and it is an unrefined cargbohydrate containing vitamins and minerals as well as calories. Dates are also high in potassium. It takes 2 dates to make 1 tablespoon of date "sugar."

Makes 1 cup
1 tablespoon contains approximately:
1 fruit exchange
40 calories

VARIATION:

DATE BUTTER: Combine 1 cup of date "sugar" with 3/4 cup water in a saucepan and bring to a boil. Reduce the heat and simmer, uncovered, for 20 minutes, or until all of the water is absorbed. Remove from the heat and cool to room temperature. Add 1/4 cup corn oil margarine and 1 teaspoon vanilla extract and blend in with a pastry blender. Store in a tightly covered container in the refrigerator. This recipe makes approximately 1-1/4 cups. One tablespoonful contains approximately 3/4 fruit exchange, 1/2 fat exchange and 53 calories. This is an excellent spread for toast, pancakes, waffles, etc.

Peach Jam

3 cups diced fresh peaches
1-1/2 teaspoons fresh lemon
    juice
1-1/2 teaspoons unflavored
    gelatin
2 teaspoons fructose

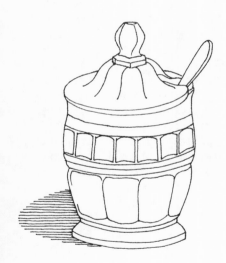

1. Put the peaches in a sauce-pan. Cover and cook over very low heat without water for about 10 minutes.
2. Remove the lid and bring the juice to the boiling point. Boil for 1 minute and remove from the heat.
3. Soften the gelatin in the lemon juice for 5 minutes. Pour some of the hot juice from the peaches into the gelatin mixture and stir until the gelatin is completely dissolved.
4. Stir the dissolved gelatin into the peaches. Allow to cool to room temperature.

Makes 3 cups
2 tablespoons contain approximately:
1/4 fruit exchange
10 calories

VARIATIONS:

WINTER PEACH JAM: Use frozen unsweetened peaches in place of the fresh peaches.

FRUIT JAM: Use other fruits as available. Check the fruit exchange list for exchange and calorie adjustments.

Banana-Peanut Pinwheels

1 banana
2 tablespoons peanut butter

1. Carefully slice the banana in half lengthwise, being careful not to break the banana halves.
2. Spread the cut side of each banana with 1/2 tablespoon of peanut butter.
3. Place the cut sides back together again, pressing firmly.
4. Slice the banana in half again, lengthwise. (The banana will now be cut into quarters, lengthwise, but 2 of them will still be "glued" together.)
5. Again spread the cut sides with peanut butter and press together, reforming the whole banana.
6. Chill slightly in the refrigerator and then slice into 1/4-inch-thick rounds.
    Banana Peanut Pinwheels are marvelous substitutes for cookies. They make wonderful after-school snacks or uniquely different garnishes for fruit salad or fruit compote.

Makes approximately 8 rounds
(pinwheels)
2 rounds (or 1/4 banana) contain
approximately:
1/2 fruit exchange
1/4 high-fat meat exchange
44 calories

VARIATIONS:

APPLE-PEANUT PINWHEELS: Cut the apple in quarters and remove the core. Spread each cut side of the apple (there will be 8 "sides") with peanut butter. Press the apple quarters back together to form a whole apple (without a core). Refrigerate until cold. Slice the apple horizontally in thin slices to make Apple-Peanut Pinwheels. One-fourth apple is only 1/4 fruit exchange, so subtract 10 calories.

● After spreading the peanut butter on either apples or bananas, lightly sprinkle the peanut butter with cinnamon before reassembling the fruit.

Banana Split with Coconut Sauce

1 envelope (1 tablespoon)
unflavored gelatin
2 tablespoons cold water
1/4 cup boiling water
2 cups non-fat milk
1 teaspoon vanilla extract
1 teaspoon coconut extract
8 bananas
Ground cinnamon for garnish

1. Soften the gelatin in the 2 tablespoons of cold water for 5 minutes. Add the boiling water and mix until the gelatin is completely dissolved.
2. Combine the dissolved gelatin with the milk and vanilla and coconut extracts and mix well. Refrigerate until jelled.
3. Cut the bananas in halves lengthwise. Place each split banana into a chilled dish.
4. Remove the jelled mixture from the refrigerator, place in a blender container and blend until it is a smooth, creamy consistency.
5. Top each split banana with 1/4 cup of the coconut sauce. Garnish with ground cinnamon.

Makes 8 servings
Each serving contains approximately:
2 fruit exchanges
1/4 non-fat milk exchange
100 calories

VARIATION:

PINEAPPLE BOATS WITH COCONUT SAUCE: Substitute 2 fresh pineapples for the bananas. Cut each pineapple lengthwise into quarters, carefully cutting through the green leaves at the top to leave a section of leaves on each pineapple quarter. Using a very sharp, small paring knife, carefully cut the pineapple from its shell. It is necessary to cut down both sides of the pineapple section. Cut the hard top core section of the pineapple off and discard it. Cut the piece of pineapple sitting on its shell in half lengthwise, then cut horizontally into bite-sized pieces. Put a pineapple quarter in each serving dish, top each pineapple quarter with the 1/4 cup of coconut sauce and sprinkle lightly with cinnamon. Subtract 1 fruit exchange and 40 calories per serving.

Note: To make a beautiful birthday dessert, place all 8 pineapple quarters on one large round serving plate with the stem ends all facing out, then place a candle in the center of each pineapple quarter.

Mediterranean Melon Balls

2/3 cup unsweetened apple juice
2 teaspoons arrowroot
1/2 teaspoon ground aniseed
4 cups melon balls (2 medium cantaloupes)

1. Combine the apple juice and arrowroot in a saucepan and stir until the arrowroot is completely dissolved.
2. Add the aniseed and mix thoroughly. Slowly bring the mixture to a boil and simmer until slightly thickened.
3. Remove the pan from the heat and cool to room temperature.
4. Combine the sauce with the melon balls and refrigerate until chilled before serving.

This is a light, low-calorie dessert that I like to serve after Moussaka for a Middle Eastern meal.

Makes 8 servings
Each serving contains approximately:
1 fruit exchange
40 calories

VARIATIONS:

● Combine the cantaloupe balls with honeydew and watermelon balls for a more colorful dessert. Check the fruit exchange list for exchange and calorie adjustments.

MIDDLE EASTERN MELON BALL SALAD: Add 1/2 cup of low-fat cottage cheese to each serving and serve on lettuce leaves. Garnish with fresh mint, if available, and serve for lunch. Add 2 low-fat meat exchanges and 110 calories per serving.

Peaches Amaretto

1 cup low-fat milk
1 tablespoon cornstarch
1 tablespoon fructose
1-1/2 teaspoons vanilla extract
3 tablespoons Amaretto liqueur
2 egg whites, at room temperature
8 medium peaches, peeled, pitted and sliced (when fresh peaches are not available, peaches canned in water or natural juice may be used)

1. Put the milk in a saucepan. Add the cornstarch and fructose and stir until the cornstarch is thoroughly dissolved.
2. Place the pan on low heat and slowly bring to a boil. Simmer, stirring constantly with a wire whisk, until slightly thickened.
3. Remove the pan from the heat and allow to cool to room temperature.
4. Add the vanilla extract and Amaretto liqueur and mix thoroughly.
5. Beat the egg whites until stiff but not dry and fold them into the sauce.
6. Divide the sliced peaches into 8 sherbet glasses or serving dishes and spoon an equal amount of the sauce over each serving.

Makes 8 servings
Each serving contains approximately:
1-1/2 fruit exchanges
60 calories

VARIATION: Substitute 1/2 teaspoon almond extract for the Amaretto. Subtract 1/4 fruit exchange and 10 calories per serving.

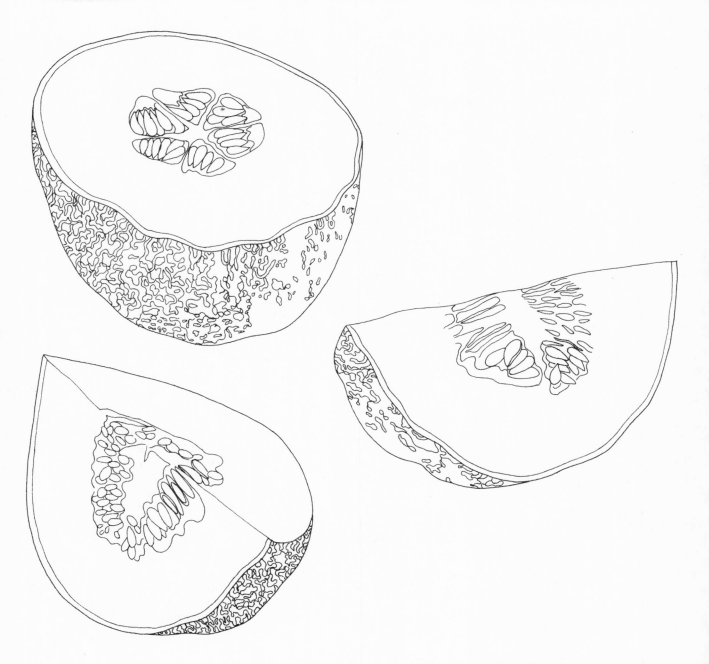

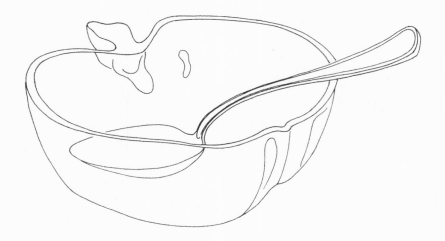

Applesauce

3 large cooking apples, peeled
   and cored
3/4 cup water
1 tablespoon fructose
1/4 teaspoon ground nutmeg
1/4 teaspoon ground
   cinnamon
1/2 teaspoon vanilla extract

1. Preheat the oven to 325°F.

2. Dice the apples into 1-inch cubes.
3. Mix together all of the remaining ingredients.
4. Put the diced apples in a glass loaf pan or baking dish (I prefer the loaf pan because the apples stay more moist). Pour the water mixture over the apples.
5. Bake, uncovered, in the preheated oven for 45 minutes. Remove from the oven and cool to room temperature. Store in a container with a tightly fitting lid in the refrigerator.

Makes 2 cups
1/2 cup contains approximately:
1-1/4 fruit exchanges
50 calories

VARIATION: If you prefer a smoothly textured applesauce, spoon the cooked apples into a blender container and blend until smooth.

Pear Sherbet

6 ripe pears
4 cups water
1/2 cup fructose

1. Peel the pears, cut them in half lengthwise and remove the cores.
2. Combine the pear halves, water and fructose in a large saucepan and bring to a boil.
3. Reduce the heat, cover and simmer for 20 minutes, or until the pears are soft. At this point the liquid should be reduced by one half. If not, remove the pears from the liquid and continue to simmer the liquid until it is reduced by one half.
4. Put all of the ingredients into a blender container and blend until completely smooth.
5. Pour the mixture into a large bowl and place it in the freezer. Every half hour, beat the mixture well, using a wire whisk. Repeat this procedure 6 times. After whipping for the last time, cover tightly or the pear sherbet will lose much of its flavor.

This sherbet is best made the day before it is to be served.

Makes 8 servings
Each serving contains approximately:
2 fruit exchanges
80 calories

VARIATION:

PEACH SHERBET: Substitute 6 medium peaches for the pears.

Frozen Blueberry "Custard"

1 envelope (1 tablespoon) unflavored gelatin
2 tablespoons cold water
1/4 cup boiling water
1 cup (1/2 pint) low-fat cottage cheese
3 tablespoons instant non-fat dry milk
2 tablespoons fructose
1-1/2 teaspoons vanilla extract
2 teaspoons lemon juice
1/4 cup cold water
1-1/2 cups frozen unsweetened blueberries, unthawed

1. Soften the gelatin in the 2 tablespoons of cold water for 5 minutes. Add the boiling water and stir until the gelatin is completely dissolved.
2. Cool the gelatin mixture for a few minutes and then pour it into a blender container.
3. Add the cottage cheese, dry milk, fructose, vanilla extract and lemon juice to the gelatin mixture and blend until completely smooth.
4. Pour the mixture into a bowl, cover and refrigerate until firm.
5. Pour the 1/4 cup of cold water in the blender container. Add the jelled cottage cheese mixture and the frozen blueberries to the blender container and blend until smooth. (It is important that the water be placed in the blender first so that the ingredients mix more easily.)

Makes 6 (1/2 cup) servings
Each serving contains approximately:
3/4 fruit exchange
3/4 low-fat meat exchange
72 calories

VARIATIONS:
• Any sliced or chopped frozen fruit may be used in place of the blueberries. Check the fruit exchange list for exchange and calorie adjustments.
• If you wish, you may use chilled unfrozen fruit, but the result will not look or taste as much like ice cream. When made with unfrozen fruit, this dish may also be used as a sauce for chopped or sliced fresh fruits.

Orange Mousse

1 envelope (1 tablespoon)
    unflavored gelatin
1/4 cup cold water
1/4 cup boiling water
1/4 cup fructose
One 6-ounce can frozen
    orange juice concentrate,
    thawed
1 egg yolk, beaten
1/4 teaspoon freshly grated
    orange rind
3 egg whites
Additional freshly grated
    orange rind for garnish

1. Soften the gelatin in the
1/4 cup of cold water for 5
minutes. Add the boiling water
and stir until the gelatin is
completely dissolved.
2. Place the fructose, orange
juice, egg yolk and gelatin
mixture into a saucepan and
cook over medium heat until
slightly thickened.

3. Remove from the heat and
stir in 1/4 teaspoon of grated
orange rind.
4. Place in a bowl in the refrigerator and chill, stirring frequently, until it is fairly firm.
5. Beat the egg whites until
stiff but not dry and fold into
the gelatin mixture.
6. Spoon the mixture into individual serving dishes and garnish with orange rind.

Makes 8 servings
Each serving contains approximately:
1-1/4 fruit exchanges
1/4 medium-fat meat exchange
69 calories

VARIATION:

ORANGE CHIFFON PIE: Pour the
mousse mixture into a pre-
baked Perfect Pie Crust, page
166. The crust will add con-
siderably to the calories (995,
to be exact), so cut the pie
into 10 servings. Each serving
contains approximately 1 fruit
exchange, 1/4 medium-fat meat
exchange, 1/2 bread exchange
and 1-1/4 fat exchanges, for a
total of 151 calories.

Lavender Soufflé

2 envelopes (2 tablespoons)
    unflavored gelatin
1 cup cold water
2 egg yolks
Two 6-ounce cans frozen
    unsweetened Concord grape
    juice concentrate, thawed
8 egg whites
1 cup evaporated skim milk,
    chilled

1. Wrap a waxed paper collar
around a 7-inch (1-quart) soufflé
dish and tape it in place
(masking tape works best). It
should rise about 3 to 5 inches
above the rim of the dish. Set
aside.
2. Soften the gelatin in the
cold water for 5 minutes.
3. Beat the egg yolks with an
electric mixer or wire whisk
until foamy. Beat in the softened
gelatin.
4. Pour the egg yolk mixture
into the top pan of a double
boiler and place over simmering
water.

5. Cook, stirring constantly, until thick enough to lightly coat a metal spoon. *Do not allow the mixture to come to a boil.*

6. Remove the pan from the heat and stir in the thawed grape juice concentrate.

7. Pour the mixture into a large mixing bowl and refrigerate until thickened to a syrupy consistency, about 45 minutes.

8. Beat the egg whites until they are stiff but not dry. Set aside.

9. In another bowl, beat the chilled evaporated milk until it has doubled in volume.

10. Fold the whipped milk gently but thoroughly into the cold grape juice mixture, using a rubber spatula.

11. Fold in the egg whites until no streaks of white show.

12. Pour the soufflé mixture into the collared soufflé dish. Refrigerate for at least 4 hours before removing the waxed paper collar and serving the soufflé.

When serving Lavender Soufflé, I like to place a very small cluster of Concord grapes or any other grapes in season on each serving plate.

Makes 16 servings
Each serving contains approximately:
1-1/2 fruit exchanges
1/2 low-fat meat exchange
88 calories

VARIATION:

COLD ORANGE SOUFFLE: Substitute two 6-ounce cans frozen unsweetened orange juice concentrate, thawed, for the frozen grape juice. Add 1/4 cup fructose to the egg whites and follow the recipe exactly. (Grape juice is sweeter than orange juice, hence the additional fructose.) Add 1/4 fruit exchange and 10 calories per serving.

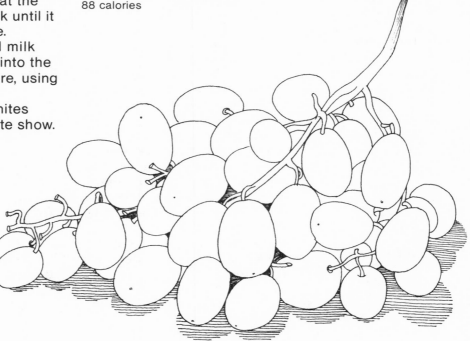

Prune Mousse

18 dried pitted prunes
3/4 cup boiling water
1 envelope (1 tablespoon)
    unflavored gelatin
2 tablespoons cold water
1/4 cup boiling water
3/4 cup low-fat cottage
    cheese
3/4 cup non-fat milk
1 teaspoon vanilla extract
1/4 teaspoon ground
    cinnamon

1. Put the pitted prunes in a large bowl and pour 3/4 cup of boiling water over them. Cover and refrigerate for 24 hours.
2. Put the prunes and all of the water from the bowl into a blender container.
3. Soften the gelatin in the cold water for 5 minutes. Add the 1/4 cup boiling water and stir until the gelatin is completely dissolved. Add the gelatin mixture and all other ingredients to the blender container.
4. Blend on high speed until frothy. Pour into a shallow rectangular or square dish. Cover tightly and refrigerate until firm.

5. To serve, cut into squares and put on plates or in sherbet glasses.
   This is just as good for breakfast as it is for dessert.

Makes 6 servings
Each serving contains approximately:
1-1/2 fruit exchanges
1/2 low-fat meat exchange
88 calories

VARIATION: Spread 6 pitted prunes, soaked in boiling water and finely chopped, in the baking dish before pouring in the mixture from the blender in step 4. Add 1/2 fruit exchange and 20 calories per serving.

Flan

4 eggs, or 1 cup liquid egg
    substitute
4 cups non-fat milk
1/4 teaspoon salt
1/4 cup fructose
1 teaspoon maple extract
1 tablespoon vanilla extract
Ground cinnamon for garnish

1. Preheat the oven to 250°F.
2. Put all of the ingredients, except the cinnamon, in a blender container and blend until smooth.

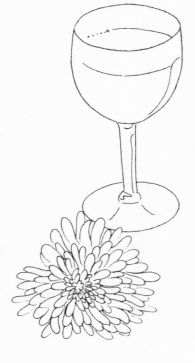

3. Pour the mixture into a 6-cup baking dish and sprinkle with ground cinnamon.

4. Set the baking dish in a shallow pan half filled with warm water and bake in the preheated oven for 2 hours, or until set.

5. Cool to room temperature and refrigerate until chilled before serving.

Flan is a traditional dessert custard served in Spain and throughout Mexico and South America. It is usually served with a caramelized sugar topping. I have used maple extract in this custard for a similar flavor.

Makes 8 servings
Each serving contains approximately:
1/2 medium-fat meat exchange
1/2 non-fat milk exchange
1/2 fruit exchange
98 calories

VARIATIONS:

EGG CUSTARD: Omit the maple extract.

EGG NOG CUSTARD: Substitute 1 teaspoon of rum extract for the maple extract. Add 1 teaspoon ground coriander in step 1. Omit the cinnamon in step 2 and use ground nutmeg in its place.

Jelled Fruitcake

1 envelope (1 tablespoon) unflavored gelatin
2 tablespoons cold water
1/4 cup boiling water
1/2 cup milk
1/2 cup unsweetened applesauce
1/2 cup raisins
1 tablespoon fructose
1/2 teaspoon ground cinnamon
1/4 teaspoon ground allspice
1/8 teaspoon ground nutmeg
1/2 teaspoon carob powder or unsweetened cocoa
1 teaspoon vanilla extract
One 8-ounce can crushed pineapple packed in natural juice, well drained
1/2 cup chopped walnuts

1. Soften the gelatin in the cold water for 5 minutes. Add the boiling water and stir until the gelatin is completely dissolved.

2. Pour the gelatin mixture and all of the other ingredients, except the crushed pineapple and walnuts, into a blender container.

3. Blend until thoroughly mixed and the raisins are coarsely chopped.

4. Pour the blended mixture into a bowl and add the crushed pineapple. Mix thoroughly.

5. Pour the mixture into an oiled 8-inch cake pan. Refrigerate until firm, several hours or overnight.

6. Before serving, preheat the oven to 350°F. Place the walnuts on a baking sheet in the center of the preheated oven for 8 to 10 minutes, or until golden brown. Watch them carefully, as they burn easily.

7. Remove the jelled fruitcake from the refrigerator and invert on a cake plate. Turn right side up and sprinkle the toasted walnuts evenly over the top of the cake.

Makes 8 servings
Each serving contains approximately:
1 fruit exchange
1/4 fat exchange
52 calories

VARIATION:

DIETER'S DREAM DESSERT Omit the raisins and the walnuts. Subtract 1/2 fruit exchange, 1/4 fat exchange and 32 calories per serving, making each serving only 20 calories for a holiday dessert!

14-Karat Cake

1 cup whole-wheat flour
1/4 cup fructose
1 teaspoon baking powder
3/4 teaspoon baking soda
1/4 teaspoon salt
1 teaspoon ground cinnamon
1/4 cup corn oil
2 eggs, lightly beaten, or
    1/2 cup liquid egg substitute
14 ounces (1-3/4 cups) scraped
    and grated carrots (3 medium
    carrots)
1 teaspoon freshly grated
    orange rind
1 large or 2 small oranges,
    peeled, seeded and very
    finely chopped
1/4 cup chopped walnuts

1. Preheat the oven to 350°F. Lightly grease the sides of an 8-1/2-inch square cake pan. Cut waxed paper to fit the bottom of the pan. (If using a Teflon pan, put waxed paper on the bottom of the pan but do not grease the sides.)
2. Combine the flour, fructose, baking powder, baking soda, salt and cinnamon in a large mixing bowl.
3. In another bowl, combine the oil and eggs and mix well.
4. Add the liquid ingredients to the dry ingredients and again mix well.
5. Add the carrots, orange rind, diced oranges and chopped walnuts and mix well.
6. Pour the batter into the cake pan and bake in the preheated oven for approximately 35 minutes, or until a wooden pick inserted in the center comes out clean.
7. Cool on a wire rack 10 minutes, then remove the cake from the pan and carefully peel off the waxed paper. Cool to room temperature and cover the cake until ready to serve so it will not dry out. If you are keeping the cake for more than a day, I suggest storing it in the refrigerator to preserve freshness.

I call this recipe "14-Karat Cake" instead of plain old carrot cake because it has 14 ounces of carrots (more carrots than most other recipes) and it also has fewer calories per serving, making it very *valuable* to the dieter!

Makes 16 servings
Each serving contains approximately:
1 fruit exchange
1 bread exchange
1/4 vegetable exchange
3/4 fat exchange
151 calories

VARIATION:

HAWAIIAN CARROT CAKE: Omit the oranges and grated orange rind and in their place add one 20-ounce can of crushed pineapple packed in natural juice, drained. Use only 1 cup of grated carrots instead of 1-3/4 cups. Follow directions exactly. Differences in exchanges and calories are negligible.

Piña Colada Cake

Cake
1-1/2 cups white pastry or
    cake flour
2 teaspoons baking powder
1/4 teaspoon salt
1/8 teaspoon cream of tartar
3 egg whites, at room
    temperature
1/4 pound (1/2 cup) corn oil
    margarine
1/2 cup fructose
One 20-ounce can crushed
    pineapple in natural juice,
    undrained

Frosting
2 cups (1 pint) low-fat cottage
    cheese
1 teaspoon vanilla extract
1 teaspoon coconut extract
4 teaspoons fructose

1. Preheat the oven to 350°F. Grease the sides of a 9-inch cake pan. Cut waxed paper to fit the bottom of the pan. (If you are using a Teflon pan, put the waxed paper on the bottom, but do not grease the sides).

2. To make the cake, sift together the flour, baking powder and salt and set aside.

3. Add the cream of tartar to the egg whites and beat until they form soft peaks. Set aside.

4. Using the same beaters, in a large mixing bowl cream together the corn oil margarine, fructose and vanilla extract until light and fluffy.

5. Add the sifted flour and 1/2 cup of the pineapple juice from the can of crushed pineapple alternately to the margarine-fructose mixture until the batter is thoroughly mixed. (Reserve the remaining pineapple juice and the crushed pineapple.)

6. Fold the beaten egg whites into the batter, being careful not to overmix.

7. Spread the batter evenly in the cake pan and bake in the preheated oven for 25 minutes, or until a wooden pick inserted in the center comes out clean.

8. While the cake is baking, make the frosting. Put the cottage cheese, vanilla and coconut extracts, fructose and remaining pineapple juice in a blender container and blend until completely smooth. Pour into a bowl, add the drained crushed pineapple and mix thoroughly with a spatula. Cover and refrigerate until the cake is cool enough to frost.

9. Cool the cake on a wire rack 10 minutes, then remove from the pan, carefully remove the waxed paper and cool to room temperature.

10. When the cake is completely cooled, slice it in half horizontally with a serrated knife, carefully dividing it into 2 equal halves. Place the bottom half, cut side up, on a cake plate and evenly spread half of the frosting on it. Place the second half of the cake, cut side down, on top of it, spreading the remaining frosting evenly over the top and sides of the cake.

11. Place the cake, covered, in the refrigerator and wait several hours before serving.

Makes 12 servings
Each serving (with frosting) contains approximately:
2 fat exchanges
1-1/2 bread exchanges
1 fruit exchange
3/4 low-fat meat exchange
277 calories
Each serving (without frosting) contains approximately:
1-1/2 bread exchanges
1 fruit exchange
145 calories

VARIATION:

BASIC WHITE CAKE: Omit the pineapple juice in the cake and replace it with 1/2 cup non-fat milk. Changes in calories and exchanges are negligible. Frost as desired or serve with fresh fruit in season (check the fruit exchange list for exchange and calorie adjustments).

Torta de Garbanzo
(Garbanzo Bean Cake)

1-1/2 cups cooked garbanzo
beans, drained (1/4 pound
dry garbanzo beans cooked
2-1/2 hours, or one 15-
ounce can)
1/2 cup non-fat milk
3 eggs, separated
1/8 teaspoon cream of tartar
1/4 cup fructose
1/8 teaspoon ground nutmeg
1/4 teaspoon ground
cinnamon
1/2 teaspoon vanilla extract
1 teaspoon rum extract

1. Preheat the oven to 350°F.
Lightly grease the sides of a
9-inch cake pan. Cut waxed
paper to fit the bottom of the
pan. (If you are using a Teflon
pan, put the waxed paper on
the bottom, but do not grease
the sides.)
2. Put the drained garbanzo
beans and the milk in a blender
container and blend until
smooth.

3. Beat the egg whites and
cream of tartar until stiff but
not dry. Set aside.
4. Beat the egg yolks until
thick. Add the fructose, nutmeg, cinnamon and vanilla and
rum extracts and mix thoroughly. Fold the beaten egg
whites into the yolk mixture.
5. Pour the batter into the
cake pan and bake in the
preheated oven for approximately 40 minutes, or until a
wooden pick inserted in the
center comes out clean.
6. Cool on a wire rack for 10
minutes, then remove the cake
from the pan and carefully
peel off the waxed paper. Cool
to room temperature, cover
and refrigerate several hours
or overnight before serving.

I like fresh pineapple with
this cake. Any fresh fruit in
season, however, is good.

Makes 12 servings
Each serving contains approximately:
1/4 medium-fat meat exchange
1/4 bread exchange
1/2 fruit exchange
57 calories

VARIATION:

BREAKFAST BEAN CAKE: Add 1/2
cup raisins in step 4. Add 1/4
fruit exchange and 10 calories
per serving.

Truly Fruity Cake

1 cup raisins
1/2 cup chopped dried apricots
1/2 cup chopped pitted dates
1 cup chopped walnuts
1 cup whole-wheat flour
1/4 cup corn oil
1 tablespoon vanilla extract
1/4 teaspoon salt
2 eggs, lightly beaten, or
1/2 cup liquid egg substitute
One 16-ounce can crushed
pineapple, packed in natural
juice, drained

1. Preheat the oven to 350°F.
2. Combine the raisins, apricots, dates, walnuts and flour
in a large bowl and mix well.
Set aside.
3. Combine all of the remaining ingredients and mix well.
4. Combine the fruit-flour mixture with the oil-egg mixture
and mix thoroughly.
5. Pour the batter into a greased
standard-sized loaf pan and
bake for 1 hour in the preheated oven.

6. Place the loaf pan on its side on a wire rack to cool to room temperature.

7. Remove the fruitcake from the pan. To serve, cut the fruitcake in half lengthwise. Slice each half into 18 pieces, making a total of 36 slices.

Makes 36 slices
Each slice contains approximately:
3/4 fruit exchange
1/2 fat exchange
1/4 bread exchange
71 calories

VARIATION:

TRULY FRUITY COOKIES: Drop by teaspoonfuls on greased baking sheets. Bake in a preheated 350°F oven for 8 to 10 minutes. Do not overcook. Makes 48 cookies. Two cookies contain approximately 1 fruit exchange, 3/4 fat exchange, 1/4 bread exchange and 92 calories.

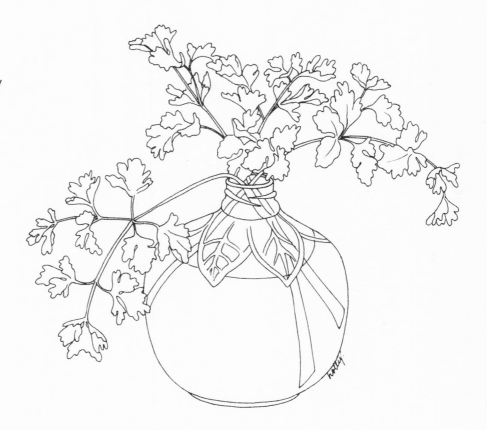

Cheesecake

2 teaspoons corn oil
   margarine
4 graham cracker squares
2 cups (1 pint) low-fat
   cottage cheese
1/4 cup fructose
2 teaspoons vanilla extract
1 teaspoon freshly grated
   lemon rind
1 teaspoon fresh lemon juice

Topping
3/4 cup sour cream
2 tablespoons fructose
1-1/2 teaspoons vanilla extract

1. Preheat the oven to 375°F.
Rub the 2 teaspoons of margarine evenly over the entire
inner surface of a 9-inch pie
plate.
2. Put the 4 graham cracker
squares in a plastic bag and
roll them with a rolling pin
until they are fine crumbs.
3. Sprinkle the crumbs evenly
over the greased pie plate,
pressing them down with your
fingertips to make certain they
stick to the surface.

4. Put the cottage cheese, fructose, vanilla extract, lemon rind
and lemon juice in a blender
container and blend until smooth.
Pour the cottage cheese mixture into the graham cracker
shell, spreading it out evenly.
5. Place in the center of the
preheated oven and cook for
15 minutes.
6. While the cake is baking,
combine all of the topping
ingredients in a mixing bowl
and mix thoroughly.
7. Remove the cheesecake
from the oven and spread the
topping evenly over the top.
Place the cake back in the
oven and continue baking for
10 more minutes.
8. Cool to room temperature
on a wire rack and refrigerate
until chilled before serving.

Makes 16 servings
Each serving contains approximately:
1/2 fat exchange
1/2 fruit exchange
71 calories

VARIATION:

BLUEBERRY CHEESECAKE: Add
1 cup frozen unsweetened blueberries, unthawed, to the topping ingredients and mix thoroughly. You are adding 2 fruit
exchanges in blueberries, which
is a negligible addition when
making 16 servings. If you
divide the cheesecake into 8
servings (142 calories each),
however, you will be adding
1/4 fruit exchange and 10
calories per serving (152 calories each).

Strawberry Chiffon Pie

1 envelope (1 tablespoon)
   unflavored gelatin
2 tablespoons cold water
1/4 cup boiling water
1 cup (1/2 pint) low-fat cottage
   cheese
3 tablespoons non-fat dry milk
   powder
3 tablespoons fructose
2 teaspoons fresh lemon juice
1-1/2 teaspoons vanilla
   extract
1-1/2 cups fresh strawberries
   or frozen unsweetened
   strawberries

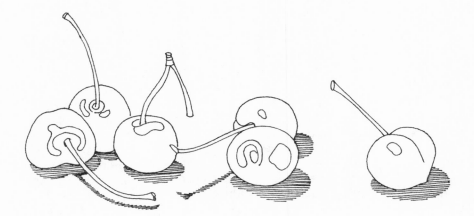

1. Soften the gelatin in the cold water for 5 minutes. Add the boiling water and stir until the gelatin is completely dissolved.

2. Reserving a few of the strawberries to place on the top of the pie for garnish, put the gelatin mixture and all of the remaining ingredients in a blender container and blend until smooth.

3. Pour into an oiled 9-inch pie plate and refrigerate until firm. If storing in the refrigerator longer than necessary for the pie to jell, be sure to cover it tightly or it will lose much of its flavor.

This dessert is best served the day it is made.

Makes 8 servings
Each serving contains approximately:
3/4 fruit exchange
1/2 low-fat meat exchange
58 calories

VARIATIONS:

BLUEBERRY CHIFFON PIE: Substitute 1-1/2 cups fresh or frozen unsweetened blueberries for the strawberries.
● Top the pie with 1/4 cup of Chiffon Pie Topping, page 163. Add 1/4 low-fat milk exchange, 1/4 fruit exchange and 42 calories per serving.
● Use a Graham Cracker Pie Crust, page 167, for the pie. Add 1 bread exchange, 1-1/2 fat exchanges and 138 calories per serving.

Chiffon Pie Topping

2 cups plain low-fat yogurt
2 teaspoons vanilla extract
1 teaspoon cherry extract
2 tablespoons fructose

1. Combine all of the ingredients and mix well.
2. Pour 1/4 cup of the topping over each serving of chiffon pie. This topping may also be used on any fresh fruit.

Makes 2 cups
1/4 cup contains approximately:
1/4 low-fat milk exchange
1/4 fruit exchange
42 calories

VARIATIONS: Try other extracts for different flavors.

Yogurt-Cheese Pie

1 Graham Cracker Pie Crust,
  page 167, baked
1 teaspoon unflavored gelatin
1 tablespoon cold water
1/4 cup boiling water
1/2 cup fructose
1 tablespoon freshly grated
  orange rind
1/4 cup fresh orange juice
3 cups Almost Ricotta Cheese,
  page 51
36 green seedless grapes,
  halved, for garnish (optional)
1 navel orange, peeled and
  sectioned, for garnish
  (optional)

1. Set the baked crust aside
to cool to room temperature.

2. Soften the gelatin in the
cold water for 5 minutes. Add
the boiling water and stir until
the gelatin is completely dissolved. Set aside.
2. Combine the fructose, orange
rind and orange juice and mix
thoroughly. Slowly add the gelatin mixture, stirring until smooth.
4. Stir the cheese into the
mixture until it is thoroughly
blended. Pour into the crust
and chill for several hours or
overnight.
5. If you are using grapes for
garnish, place the halves, cut
side down, around the outer
edge of the pie and arrange
the orange sections in the
middle of the pie.

Makes 16 servings
Each serving (with garnish)
  contains approximately:
3/4 fruit exchange
3/4 non-fat milk exchange
1/2 bread exchange
3/4 fat exchange
159 calories

VARIATIONS:

● Garnish with strawberries
and mint instead of grapes
and orange sections. Check
the fruit exchange list for exchange and calorie differences.
● Instead of using a Graham
Cracker Pie Crust, oil the pie
plate or spray it with non-stick
coating and sprinkle lightly with
the crumbs from 2 crushed
graham cracker squares. This
will eliminate the 3/4 fat exchange and the 1/2 bread
exchange and about 60 calories per serving.

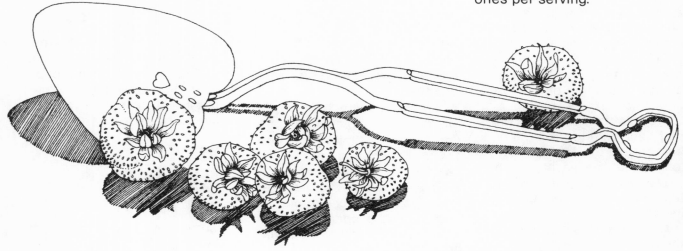

Pineapple Pumpkin Pie

1 Graham Cracker Pie Crust and Topping, page 167, baked
2 envelopes (2 tablespoons) unflavored gelatin
3 tablespoons cold water
1/4 cup boiling water
One 16-ounce can cooked pumpkin
One 8-ounce can crushed pineapple in natural juice, undrained
4 dates, pitted and chopped
1 cup non-fat milk
1-1/2 teaspoons ground cinnamon
1/4 teaspoon ground ginger
1/8 teaspoon ground cloves
2 teaspoons vanilla extract

1. Set the baked crust aside to cool to room temperature.
2. Soften the gelatin in the cold water for 5 minutes. Add the boiling water and stir until the gelatin is completely dissolved.
3. Put the gelatin mixture and all of the remaining ingredients in a blender container and blend until smooth and frothy.
4. Allow the mixture to stand until slightly thickened before pouring into the baked pie shell.

5. Sprinkle the reserved graham cracker crumbs from the pie crust recipe over the top of the pie and chill for at least 3 hours before serving.

Makes 8 servings
Each serving contains approximately:
1-1/4 bread exchanges
1-1/2 fat exchanges
3/4 fruit exchange
186 calories

VARIATION:

APPLESAUCE PUMPKIN PIE: Substitute 1 cup applesauce for the crushed pineapple.

Grasshopper Pie

1 Graham Cracker Pie Crust and Topping, page 167, baked
1 envelope (1 tablespoon) unflavored gelatin
2 tablespoons cold water
1/4 cup boiling water
2 cups non-fat milk
1-1/2 teaspoons vanilla extract
1/4 teaspoon mint extract
1 teaspoon liquid chlorophyll
2 tablespoons fructose

1. Allow the crust to cool to room temperature.
2. Soften the gelatin in the cold water. Add the boiling water and stir until the gelatin is completely dissolved.

3. Add the non-fat milk to the gelatin mixture and mix thoroughly. Place in the refrigerator for about 30 minutes, or until the mixture starts to thicken.
4. Remove the gelatin mixture from the refrigerator and pour into a blender container. Add the vanilla extract, mint extract, chlorophyll and fructose and blend until foamy.
5. Pour into the cooled pie crust. Sprinkle the reserved cookie crumbs evenly over the top and place the pie in the refrigerator to chill for at least 3 hours before serving. If possible, make a day ahead of time.

Makes 8 servings
Each serving contains approximately:
1/4 fruit exchange
1 bread exchange
1/4 non-fat milk exchange
1-1/2 fat exchanges
168 calories

VARIATION: Substitute 1 Chocolate Graham Cracker Pie Crust and Topping, page 167, for the pie crust.

Peachy Cream Pie

1 Graham Cracker Pie Crust,
  page 167, baked
1 envelope (1 tablespoon)
  unflavored gelatin
2 tablespoons cold water
1/4 cup boiling water
3/4 cup low-fat cottage
  cheese
1/4 cup low-fat milk
1-1/2 teaspoons vanilla
  extract
1/2 teaspoon almond extract
2 tablespoons fructose
2 cups finely chopped
  peaches (3 large peaches)
Ground cinnamon for garnish

1. Set the baked crust aside
to cool to room temperature.
2. Soften the gelatin in the
cold water for 5 minutes. Add
the boiling water and stir until
the gelatin is completely dissolved.

3. Put the gelatin mixture in a
blender container, add all of
the remaining ingredients, except the peaches, and blend
thoroughly.
4. Add 1/2 cup of the peaches
and blend until smooth. Pour
the mixture into a bowl.
5. Add the remaining peaches
and mix well. Pour the mixture
into the pie crust, sprinkle with
cinnamon and refrigerate until
firm.

Makes 8 servings
Each serving contains approximately:
1 bread exchange
1-1/2 fat exchanges
3/4 fruit exchange
1/2 low-fat meat exchange
196 calories

VARIATIONS:

PEACHY RUM CREAM PIE: Substitute 1/2 teaspoon rum extract for the almond extract.

● Omit the Graham Cracker
Pie Crust. Subtract 1 bread
exchange, 1-1/2 fat exchanges
and 138 calories per serving.

Perfect Pie Crust

1 cup whole-wheat pastry flour
1/4 teaspoon salt
1/4 cup corn oil
3 tablespoons ice water

1. Preheat the oven to 375°F.
2. Combine the flour and salt
in a 9-inch pie pan and mix
well.
3. Measure the oil in a large
measuring cup. Add the water
to the oil and mix well, using a
fork.
4. Slowly add the liquid to the
flour mixture in the pie pan,
mixing it with the same fork.
Continue mixing until all ingredients are well blended. Press
onto the bottom and sides with
your fingertips. Make sure that
the crust covers the entire inner
surface of the pie pan evenly.

5. Prick the bottom of the crust in several places with a fork and place in the preheated oven for 20 to 25 minutes, or until a golden brown. (If the recipe doesn't call for a pre-baked crust, omit this step.)

I feel sure that you'll agree with me that this is the simplest way to make pie crust!

Makes one 9-inch pie crust
  (8 servings)
Each serving contains approximately:
3/4 bread exchange
1-1/2 fat exchanges
121 calories
1 pie crust contains approximately:
6-1/2 bread exchanges
1-1/2 fat exchanges
995 calories

VARIATION:

PERFECT BRAN PIE CRUST: Replace 1/4 cup of whole-wheat pastry flour with 1/4 cup of unprocessed wheat bran. Subtract 1/2 bread exchange and 35 calories per crust.

Graham Cracker Pie
Pie Crust and Topping

16 graham cracker squares
4 tablespoons corn oil
  margarine, at room
  temperature

1. Preheat the oven to 375°F.
2. Put the graham cracker squares in a large plastic bag and crush with a rolling pin until they are fine crumbs.
3. Put the crumbs in a bowl and add the margarine. Using a pastry blender or a fork, mix the crumbs with the margarine until completely mixed and the consistency of a stiff dough. Reserve 2 tablespoons of this mixture to use later.
4. Place the remaining mixture in a 9- or 10-inch pie plate and, with your fingertips, press out evenly over the entire inner surface of the pie plate.
5. Place the reserved 2 tablespoons of the mixture in another baking dish to be baked at the same time as the crust.
6. Place both the pie crust and the reserved crumbs in the preheated oven and bake for 8 minutes.

7. Cool the pie crust to room temperature before adding a filling. Use the 2 tablespoons of the mixture for sprinkling over the top of the filling.

Makes 1 pie crust (8 servings)
Each serving contains approximately:
1 bread exchange
1-1/2 fat exchanges
138 calories
1 pie crust contains approximately:
8 bread exchanges
12 fat exchanges
995 calories

VARIATIONS:

CINNAMON GRAHAM CRACKER PIE CRUST AND TOPPING: Add 1/2 teaspoon ground cinnamon to the crumbs and mix thoroughly before adding the margarine.

CHOCOLATE GRAHAM CRACKER PIE CRUST AND TOPPING: Omit 2 graham cracker squares from the recipe and add 2-1/2 tablespoons unsweetened cocoa.

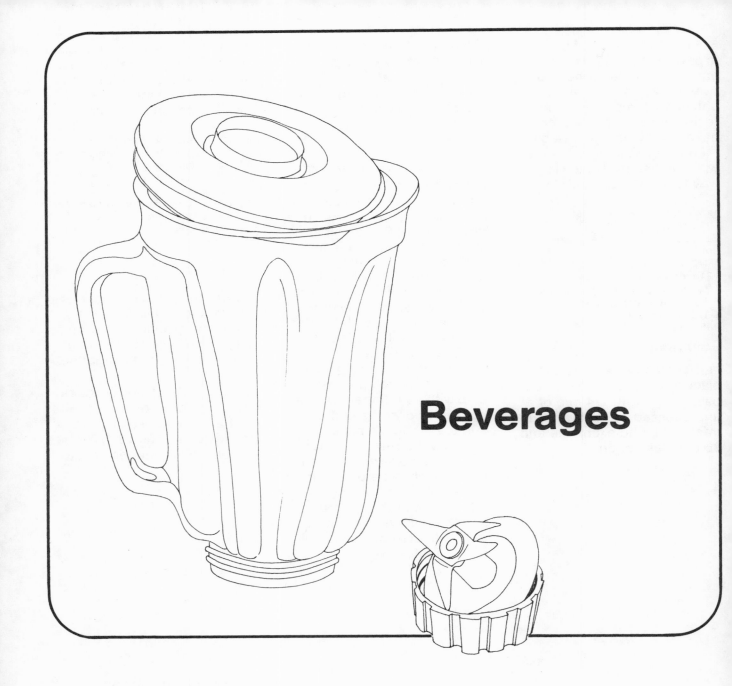

Beverages

Beverages

Beverages, like soups, can be served hot or cold, calorie free or calorie packed. In this section you will find a little bit of everything.

The only beverage recipe in this section that also appears in *The Calculating Cook* is my Counterfeit Cocktail. I have included it again because it is still my favorite cocktail party beverage.

Counterfeit Cocktail

Soda water or Perrier water
  (enough to fill a tall glass)
Ice cubes
1/2 fresh lime
Dash of Angostura bitters

1. Pour the soda water over ice in a tall glass.
2. Add the juice of 1/2 lime and a dash of bitters. Stir and serve.

Makes 1 serving
Free food
Calories negligible

VARIATION:

WOOSTER WONDER: Use a dash of Worcestershire sauce in place of the bitters and substitute a dash of lemon juice for the lime. Use a lemon slice or twist for garnish. Calories are still negligible. This cocktail decidedly falls in the "don't knock it until you've tried it" category. I discovered it one day by inadvertently adding Worcestershire sauce instead of bitters, and liked it so much that I now occasionally do it on purpose.

Cold "Gin" Sling
(Just the Juniper Berries!)

4 cups water
1/4 cup juniper berries
1 tablespoon fresh lemon
  juice
3 tablespoons fructose
Ice cubes

1. Bring the water and juniper berries to a boil in a saucepan, reduce the heat, cover and simmer for 1 hour.
2. Remove from the heat and add the lemon juice and fructose. Mix thoroughly and cool to room temperature.
3. Refrigerate, covered, for at least 24 hours before serving.
4. To serve, strain and serve over ice in chilled glasses.

This is similar to an unusual and refreshing beverage served at The Prophet Vegetarian Restaurant in San Diego. Every time I have it I like it better, so I decided to include it in this book.

Makes 4 servings
Each serving contains approximately:
3/4 fruit exchange
30 calories

VARIATION:

THE REAL THING SLING: Stir in 1 ounce of gin before serving. Check the alcoholic beverage list for the calories, depending upon the proof of the gin (67 to 83 calories per ounce).

Margarita Fingida

(Fake Margarita)

1-1/2 cups soda water or
   Perrier water
2 tablespoons fresh lime juice
1 tablespoon fructose
1 egg white (dip the egg in
   boiling water for 30 seconds
   before breaking)
1/2 cup crushed ice
Coarse salt
Ice cubes
Lime slices for garnish

1. Pour the soda water into a
blender container. Add the lime
juice, fructose, egg white and
crushed ice and blend until
frothy.
2. Rub lime around the rims of
4 chilled glasses. Dip the rim
of each glass into the salt. Fill
each glass with ice cubes, and
then fill with the frothy margarita
mixture and garnish with a
slice of lime.

Makes 4 servings
Each serving contains approximately:
1/4 fruit exchange
10 calories

VARIATION:

STRAWBERRY MARGARITA: Add
3/4 cup frozen unsweetened
strawberries and 1 more tablespoon fructose to the blender
container in step 1. Add 1/2
fruit exchange and 20 calories
per serving.

Sparkling Apple Aperitif

2 cups cold unsweetened
   apple juice
2 cups soda water or Perrier
   water
Apple slices for garnish
   (optional)
Cinnamon sticks for garnish
   (optional)

1. Combine the cold apple juice
and soda water, mixing well.
2. Serve in chilled wine or
champagne glasses. Garnish
with apple slices and cinnamon
sticks, if desired.

Makes 8 (1/2 cup) servings
Each serving contains approximately:
1/2 fruit exchange
20 calories

VARIATION:

CHAMPAGNE APPLE APERITIF:
Substitute 2 cups of cham-
pagne for the sparkling water.
Add 50 calories per serving.

Paradise Punch

1 cup fresh orange juice
One 8-ounce can crushed
   pineapple in natural juice,
   undrained
1 banana, peeled and sliced
1 cup non-fat milk
1 tablespoon fructose
1 teaspoon vanilla extract
1/2 teaspoon coconut extract
1/2 cup crushed ice
Fresh mint sprigs for garnish
   (optional)

1. Combine all of the ingredients, except the mint, in a
blender container and blend
until smooth and frothy.
2. Pour into 4 chilled glasses
and garnish with fresh mint, if
available.

Makes 4 servings
Each serving contains approximately:
2 fruit exchanges
1/4 non-fat milk exchange
100 calories

VARIATION:

PARTY PARADISE PUNCH: Add rum
to taste to the blender mixture.
Check the alcoholic beverages
list for the calories, depending
upon the quantity used and
the proof of the rum. Alcohol
has "empty" calories (no nutritional value), so there is no
exchange factor.

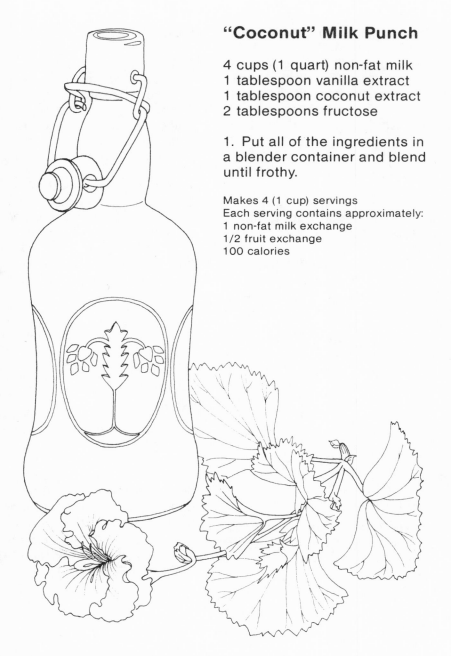

"Coconut" Milk Punch

4 cups (1 quart) non-fat milk
1 tablespoon vanilla extract
1 tablespoon coconut extract
2 tablespoons fructose

1. Put all of the ingredients in a blender container and blend until frothy.

Makes 4 (1 cup) servings
Each serving contains approximately:
1 non-fat milk exchange
1/2 fruit exchange
100 calories

VARIATION:

PINA COLADA PUNCH: Substitute 2 cups unsweetened pineapple juice for 2 cups of the milk. Add 1-1/2 fruit exchanges, subtract 1/2 non-fat milk exchange and add 20 calories per serving.

Pineapple Punch

1/2 cup unsweetened
   pineapple juice
1 cup diced cantaloupe
3 ice cubes
Ice cubes for serving

1. Put all of the ingredients in a blender container and blend until smooth.
2. Serve over ice cubes in tall glasses.

Makes 2 servings
Each serving contains approximately:
1 fruit exchange
40 calories

VARIATION:

SPARKLING PINEAPPLE PUNCH: Add soda water or Perrier water to the ingredients in the blender container (as much as you want) to make the drink even taller and add some sparkle.

Applesauce Shake

1 cup non-fat milk
1 cup unsweetened
   applesauce
1/4 teaspoon ground
   cinnamon
1/2 teaspoon vanilla extract

1. Put all of the ingredients in a blender container and blend until smooth and frothy.
2. Serve in chilled glasses.

Makes 2 servings
Each serving contains approximately:
1 fruit exchange
1/2 non-fat milk exchange
80 calories

VARIATIONS:

HOT APPLE TODDY: Serve hot in mugs garnished with cinnamon sticks. Be careful not to boil while heating. This is a marvelous breakfast beverage to serve in place of hot chocolate.

APPLESAUCE WHIP: Add 1 envelope (1 tablespoon) unflavored gelatin (softened in 2 tablespoons of cold water for 5 minutes and dissolved in 1/4 cup boiling water) to the blender container. Pour into a bowl and refrigerate until firm. Makes 4 servings. Each serving contains approximately 1/2 fruit exchange, 1/4 non-fat milk exchange and 40 calories. This is a delicious low-calorie dessert.

Fresh Grapefruit Fizz

1 cup fresh grapefruit juice
2 cups soda water or Perrier
   water
Ice cubes
4 cinnamon sticks for garnish
   (optional)

1. Combine the grapefruit juice and soda water and mix well.
2. Fill 4 chilled glasses with ice and pour 3/4 cup of the fizz in each glass.
3. Garnish with a cinnamon stick, if desired.

   This is a particularly refreshing drink during the holidays, when most people are eating more rich food than usual.

Makes 4 servings
Each serving contains approximately:
1/2 fruit exchange
20 calories

VARIATION:

FRESH ORANGE FIZZ: Substitute orange juice for the grapefruit juice.

Peanut Butter Punch

2 cups non-fat milk
1/4 cup unhomogenized
   smooth peanut butter
2 tablespoons fructose
2 teaspoons vanilla extract
1 cup crushed ice
Ground cinnamon for garnish

1. Put all of the ingredients, except the cinnamon, in a blender container and blend until smooth and creamy.
2. Pour into 4 chilled glasses and sprinkle the top of each glass lightly with ground cinnamon.

Makes 4 servings
Each serving contains approximately:
1/2 non-fat milk exchange
1/2 high-fat meat exchange
1/2 fruit exchange
108 calories

VARIATIONS:

● Omit the ice, heat the punch and serve hot for breakfast instead of cocoa.

PEANUT BUTTER PUNCHER: Add dark rum to taste to the blender mixture. Check the alcoholic beverage list for calories, which will depend upon the quantity and proof of the rum.

Hot Spiced Tomato Juice

One 46-ounce can tomato
  juice
2 teaspoons Worcestershire
  sauce
3/4 teaspoon garlic salt
1/4 teaspoon crushed dried
  basil
1/4 teaspoon crushed dried
  oregano
3 drops Tabasco sauce

1. Put all of the ingredients in
a large saucepan. Bring to a
boil over low heat.
2. Pour the hot juice into mugs
and serve as the first course
to your guests before they
come to the buffet table.

Makes 12 (1/2 cup) servings
Each serving contains approximately:
1 vegetable exchange
25 calories

VARIATION:

COLD SPICED TOMATO JUICE:
Chill the spiced tomato juice
and serve it cold.

Jamaican Coffee

4 cups (1 quart) hot freshly
  made strong coffee
2 tablespoons fructose
2 teaspoons rum extract
1/2 cup Whipped "Cream,"
  page 43

1. Combine the coffee, fructose
and rum extract and mix well.
2. Pour into 4 mugs. Spoon 2
tablespoons of the cream on
top of each serving.

Makes 4 servings
Each serving contains approximately:
1/2 fruit exchange
20 calories

VARIATIONS:

IRISH COFFEE: Substitute 2 teaspoons brandy extract for the
rum extract.

● Use real rum to taste in the
Jamaican Coffee and real Irish
whiskey to taste in the Irish
Coffee. Check the alcoholic
beverage list for calories, which
will depend upon the quantity
and proof of the liquor.

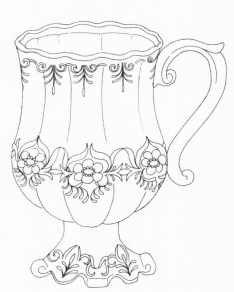

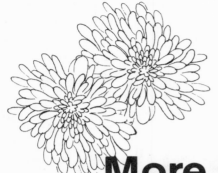

More Calculated Hints

Saturated Fat Control

To lower the amount of saturated fat in your diet, apply the following rules to your diet program:
1. Use liquid vegetable oils and margarines that are high in polyunsaturated fats in place of butter. Two of the best oils for this purpose are safflower oil and corn oil.
2. Do not use coconut oil or chocolate. Many non-dairy creamers and sour-cream substitutes contain coconut oil. Use coconut extract and powdered cocoa.
3. Use non-fat milk, or low-sodium low-fat milk if on a low-sodium diet.
4. Avoid commercial ice cream.
5. Limit the amount of beef, lamb and pork in your diet to four or five times a week and eat fish, chicken, veal and white meat of turkey in their place.
6. Buy lean cuts of meat and trim all visible fat from them before cooking.

Cholesterol Control

To lower the amount of cholesterol in your diet, apply the following restrictions to your diet program:
1. Limit or avoid egg yolks.
2. Limit shellfish such as oysters, clams, scallops, lobster, shrimp and crab.
3. Limit or avoid organ meats of all animals, such as liver, heart, kidney, sweetbreads and brains.

Sodium Control

1. The first and most obvious way of controlling the amount of sodium in the diet is to avoid the addition of ordinary table salt (sodium chloride), to already prepared foods. One teaspoon of salt contains 2,200 milligrams of sodium!

2. If you are on a sodium-restricted diet and must greatly reduce the amount of sodium in the diet, the milligrams of sodium in the serving portions of all foods can be found in the exchange lists on pages 16 through 27.

3. *Low-sodium Milk* It is also possible to reduce sodium intake by using low-sodium milk in place of regular milk both for drinking and cooking.

4. *Low-sodium Baking Powder* Regular baking powder contains 40 milligrams of sodium per teaspoon, while low-sodium baking powder contains only 1 milligram per teaspoon. When using the latter, however, you will need to add half again as much to a recipe (50 percent more) as you would if using regular baking powder. If you are unable to buy low-sodium baking powder, ask your druggist to make it for you using the following formula:

Cornstarch: 56.0 grams
Potassium bitartrate: 112.25 grams
Potassium bicarbonate: 79.5 grams
Tartaric acid: 15.0 grams

5. *Potassium Bicarbonate* Potassium bicarbonate is substituted for baking soda in the low-sodium diet. Baking soda is sodium bicarbonate and contains 1,232 milligrams of sodium per teaspoon, while potassium bicarbonate contains no sodium. Most low-sodium cookbooks tell you to use potassium bicarbonate in the same amount as you would baking soda. I have found that it has a definite aftertaste when used in that quantity, and that half as much will give you the desired results in texture without the unpleasant flavor.

6. *Drinking Water* Check with your local water district about the sodium content of your drinking water. If there are more than 30 milligrams of sodium per quart, it is advisable to use distilled water for both drinking and cooking.

7. To heighten flavor in the absence of added salt, fresh lemon juice in combination with a small amount of fructose and a greater amount of herbs or spices will produce the desired result.

Eggs

When using raw eggs or raw egg whites, it is important to coddle or dip the whole egg (in the shell) in boiling water for 30 seconds before using it. The reason for this is that avedin, a component of raw egg whites, is believed to block the absorption of biotin, one of the water-soluble vitamins. Avedin is extremely sensitive to heat and coddling the egg inactivates it.

Fructose

As June Biermann and Barbara Toohey point out in *The Diabetic's Total Health Book,* fructose is not the "free lunch" diabetics have been looking for. I agree with them that "a tablespoon of fructose does not seem a good trade for a fresh, juicy peach or ten large, sweet cherries or a small, crunchy apple." One tablespoonful of it does count as one fruit exchange in the diabetic diet, however, and as much as I love fresh fruit, I'm willing to make the trade once in a while in order to have a special dessert that requires fructose to make it taste just right.

I do not believe in the use of

artificial substitutes. I see no reason for eating unnecessary chemicals. Of all the natural sweeteners I think fructose is by far the best. It is approximately one and one-half times sweeter than sucrose (ordinary table sugar) and therefore you use less of it in most foods (fructose is sweeter when cold than when hot, so there is no real advantage in its level of sweetness when used in beverages such as hot coffee or tea). The fact that fructose is much sweeter than ordinary table sugar automatically reduces the calories and grams of carbohydrate in many recipes.

Fructose also heightens natural fruit flavor and makes fruit seem more ripe than it is. Many people who have always used salt on melon find that just a pinch of fructose is an even greater flavor enhancer. This is particularly important for people on sodium-restricted diets.

Fructose is an excellent flavor heightener in vegetable preparations in place of salt. It may also be used in small amounts in marinades, even when the desired effect is not sweetness. This is because, in the absence of salt, fructose serves as a flavor heightener and sharpens the taste of the other ingredients.

But—no fructose binges please. As June and Barbara say: It's not a free lunch! Remember that one tablespoon of fructose counts as one fruit exchange.

Wines

Never use wines for cooking that are labeled "cooking wine," because they contain salt. In fact, the term "cooking wine" goes back to a time when the wine for kitchen use was salted to prevent the cook from drinking it!

Menus

During the seven years I have been doing menus for *Diabetes Forecast* magazine, I have had many requests from readers for back issues containing specific menus and recipes. When I learned that many of the back issues are no longer available, I decided to include some of the menus and the recipes that go with them in this book. Some of the recipes have been improved and updated from the original versions.

When you are doing your own menu planning, it is important to make certain that the menu "works" from a traditional standpoint. For example, if you are serving a Mexican entrée, you would not want to do an Italian antipasto as a first course any more than you would serve gazpacho before lasagna. Remember too that appearance is important. The combination of the colors on a plate and the size and texture of the foods served all contribute to the overall appearance of the meal. Imagine how drab a plate of broiled chicken with mashed potatoes and cauliflower would look. The same plate would be gorgeous if the chicken were served with a colorful rice pilaf and steamed green broccoli. If you are serving a casserole with chopped meat as an entrée, then don't serve chopped vegetables with it. Foods should all be of varying sizes, shapes and colors. Garnishes are very important for a finished, professional presentation. Use your imagination. It is fun to garnish summer plates with flowers as well as fruits and vegetables.

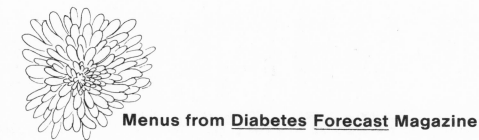

Menus from <u>Diabetes</u> <u>Forecast</u> Magazine

EASTER BRUNCH
Fresh Mint Fizz
Curried Easter Eggs
Pineapple Ham
Orange Bread

SUMMER PICNIC
Raw vegetable sticks
  with Sauer Family Cream
Marinated Carrot Sticks
Chicken Salad Sandwiches
Chopped Ham Sandwiches
Oriental-Style Deviled Eggs
Fresh fruit
"Coconut" Milk Punch

MEXICAN FIESTA
Margarita Fingida
Gazpacho Salad
Toasted Tortilla Chips
Enchiladas de Pollo
Torta de Garbanzo
Fresh fruit

INDIAN VEGETARIAN MENU
Cold Curried Grapefruit Soup
Palak Paneer
Masala Dosa
Sliced tomatoes
Herbed tea

PARTY BUFFET
Hot Spiced Tomato Juice
Celery Victor
French Dressing Marinade
Turkey Stroganoff
Whole-Wheat Noodles
Herbed Carrots and Parsley
Jelled Fruitcake

**'TIS THE SEASON
TO BE JOLLY**
Sherried Pea Soup
Cornish Game Hens à l'Orange
Vegetable Dressing
Christmas Rice Pilaf
Pineapple Pumpkin Pie

HOLIDAY DINNER
Relish Tray: celery hearts,
  radish roses, carrot sticks
Chicken Consommé
Cranberry-Apple Holiday
  Wreath Salad
Roast Turkey with Mushroom
  Gravy
Almond-Rice Dressing
Pumpkin Puff in Orange Cups
Bouillon-Baked Onions
French-cut green beans
Grasshopper Pie

**CHANUKAH (HANUKKAH)
FEAST**
Fruit juice cocktail
Eggplant Appetizer
Chicken-Mushroom Soup
Candle Salad
Roast Chicken
Potato Latkes with Applesauce
Green beans
Cheesecake

Curing Your Iron Skillets

The purpose of "curing" your iron skillets is to use them for browning meat, cooking pancakes, omelettes and crêpes, etc., without added fat. I prefer a cured iron skillet to Teflon because it's better for browning and I don't have to worry about scratching it.

To cure your new iron skillet, or your grandmother's old one, put several tablespoons of oil in it. Put it on moderate heat and when it starts to get hot, tilt it from side to side until the oil coats the entire inner surface of the skillet. Continue heating the skillet until it gets so hot it starts to smoke. Then turn the heat off and cool the skillet. When it's cool enough to handle, wipe all the oil out of it with paper towels. Repeat this process three or four times and you have a cured pan.

Never wash a cured pan with water. When you are through with it each time, wipe it out with oil. If anything is stuck on the bottom, rub it off with salt. If you *have* to wash it with water or if you have used it for cooking liquids, all is not lost. Don't throw the pan away, just cure it again!

Dr. James Briggs, at that time president of the California Nutrition Council, was quoted in the *San Diego Union* as saying that the amount of dietary iron in foods cooked in iron cookware is significantly higher than those cooked in aluminum, glass or coated cookware. He said: "There is something in the way women used to cook. They stirred a lot and actually scraped a little iron off the skillet into the food. That is the kind of iron the body can use." I was so pleased to learn that the skillets I had been using for years were good for my health as well as my cooking!

Using Herbs and Spices

We have only four basic tastes. They are, in order, from the tip of the tongue back: sweet, salt, sour and bitter. All other "tastes" are actually smells. If you don't believe me, hold your nose the next time you eat and you will find that you don't "taste" anything! Or remember back to the time you had a bad cold and couldn't "taste" anything.

Because our sense of smell is so important to the flavor of our food, herbs and spices can play a very important role in making foods taste better. Also, by using herbs and spices imaginatively, you can create new and exciting flavors in your own cooking and baking.

Fresh herbs and spices are wonderful and always add a glamorous touch as well as a delightful flavor. *Always* use fresh parsley. Dried parsley, in my opinion, tastes exactly like hay, and tends to ruin rather than enhance flavor. Try growing at least some of your own herbs if you can. It's fun to be able to go right outside your back door or to your window sill to pick your herbs.

When using dry herbs and spices, always crush them well, using a mortar and pestle, before adding them to your recipe. This is very important because it releases much more of their aroma and thus increases their flavor. You can tell when you have crushed them enough because the odor of the herb or spice will be markedly increased.

The following list of herbs and spices gives all of their traditional uses, as well as some rather unusual ones. Not only will using more herbs and spices in your cooking increase the flavor range of your menus; it will also make it possible to cut calories by using less margarine and fewer nuts, seeds and other high-calorie ingredients used to give flavor to foods. This is particularly important in the diabetic diet where fat exchanges are precious!

ALLSPICE: Fruit, sweet potatoes, squash, eggs, fish, pot roast.

ANISEED: Cheese, beverages, cookies, cakes, breads, fish, stew, fruit dishes.

BASIL: All vegetables, fish, meat and poultry, egg dishes, sauces and salad dressings, all Italian dishes in combination with oregano.

BAY LEAF: Roasts, stews, soups, marinades, poultry dressings, chowders.

CARDAMOM: Fruit soups, squash, baked goods, sweet potatoes.

CAYENNE PEPPER: Sauces, vegetables, cheese, eggs, fish, chicken, pizza, spaghetti, meat dishes.

CELERY SEED: Soups, stews, meat loaf, egg dishes, breads, rolls, stuffings, potato salad, tomatoes, many other vegetables.

CHILI POWDER: Corn, bean casseroles, cheese, marinades, chicken, meat loaf, stews, egg dishes, tomato or barbecue sauces, dips.

CINNAMON: Lamb and beef stews, roast lamb, chicken, pork, ham, beverages, bakery products, fruits.

CLOVES: Glazed pork and beef, tomatoes, sweet potatoes, carrots, green beans, marinades for meats, pot roast, meat sauces, stuffings, fish, baked goods, fruits; for studding ham.

CORIANDER: Meat, poultry, stuffings, curry sauces, fruit, barbecue sauces, fruit salads, custards, marinated bean salads.

CUMIN: Chili, omelets, salad dressings.

CURRY POWDER: Curried beef, poultry and fish dishes, eggs, dried beans, fruit, dips, breads, salad dressings, marinades.

DILL SEED AND DILL WEED: Sauces, green beans, egg dishes, fish, chicken, breads.

FENNEL: Sauerkraut, breads, cakes, cookies, egg dishes, fish, stews, marinades for meats, vegetables, cheese, baked and stewed apples.

GARLIC: Meat, poultry, fish, stews, marinades, tomato dishes, soups, dips, sauces, salads, salad dressings, etc.!

GINGER: Baked and stewed fruits, vegetables, baked goods, poultry, fish, meat, beverages, soups, Oriental dishes.

JUNIPER BERRIES: Venison, game or rabbit, stew, hot and cold drinks.

MACE: Fruits, meat loaf, fish, poultry, chowder, vegetables.

MARJORAM: Soups, breads, egg dishes, spaghetti, pizza, broccoli, mushrooms, squash, peas, cauliflower, carrots, tomato dishes, meat, poultry, fish.

MINT: Sauces for lamb and poultry, punches, tea, dessert sauces, vegetables.

DRY MUSTARD: Vegetables, fish, meat, poultry, salad dressings, egg dishes, cheese dishes.

MUSTARD SEED: Corned beef, cole slaw, potato salad, boiled cabbage, pickles, sauerkraut.

NUTMEG: Hot beverages, puddings, fish, meat, poultry, fruits, baked goods, eggs, vegetables, pickles.

ONION POWDER: Breads, egg dishes, rice dishes, cheese dishes, stuffings, vegetables, salads, fish, meat, poultry, stews, soups, dips.

OREGANO: Fish, meat, poultry, all vegetables, stuffings, cheese dishes, egg dishes, barbecue sauce, chili con carne, pizza, pasta sauces, tomatoes.

PAPRIKA: Fish, meat, poultry, egg dishes, cheese dishes; for adding color to colorless vegetables and for sprinkling on casseroles for garnish.

PARSLEY: Salads, broiled meat, fish, and poultry, soups, coleslaw, breads, tomato sauces, meat sauces; for garnish on many dishes.

PEPPER (BLACK): Fish, meat, poultry, eggs, vegetables, pickles, etc.

PEPPER (RED): Barbecued beef and pork, tamale pie, dips, curried dishes, spaghetti sauce, vegetables, poultry, pickles, sauces, cheese dishes, soups, meats.

PEPPER (WHITE): Vegetables, white and light meats, poultry and fish.

POULTRY SEASONING: Stuffings, poultry, veal, meat loaf, chicken soup.

ROSEMARY: Soups, stews, marinades, potatoes, cauliflower, spinach, mushrooms, turnips, fruits, breads, fish, meat, poultry.

SAFFRON: Chicken, seafood, rice.

SAGE: Sauces, soups, chowders, marinades, onions, tomatoes, cheese dishes, egg dishes, stuffings for meat, fish and poultry.

SAVORY: Tomatoes, seafood.

TARRAGON: Casseroles, marinades, sauces and salad dressings, egg dishes, fish, meat, poultry.

THYME: Fish, meat, poultry, vegetables, rice.

TURMERIC: Chutney, pickles, rice dishes, egg dishes, curried meat, fish, poultry, breads, cakes.

Kitchen Vocabulary

BAKE Cook in heated oven.

BARBECUE Cook over hot coals.

BASTE Spoon liquid over food while it is cooking as directed, or use a baster.

BEAT Using egg beater or electric mixer, beat to add air and increase volume.

BLANCH Dip quickly into boiling water. Usually refers to fruits and vegetables. When blanching nuts, cover shelled nuts with cold water and bring to a boil. Remove from heat and drain. Slip skins from nuts.

BLEND Combine two or more ingredients well; often used when referring to an electric blender.

BLEND UNTIL FROTHY Blend until foamy and the volume is almost doubled by the addition of air.

BOIL Cook food in liquid in which bubbles constantly rise to the surface and break. At sea level, water boils at 212°F.

BONE Remove all bones; usually refers to roasts and poultry.

BRAISE Brown meat well on all sides, then add a small amount of water or other liquid. Cover and simmer over low heat or place in a moderate oven and cook until tender or as recipe directs.

BROIL Cook under broiler at designated distance from heat.

BROWN Brown in oven under a broiler or in a heavy iron skillet to desired color.

CHILL Place in refrigerator until cold.

CHOP Using a large chopping knife, hold point end down with one hand and use the other hand to chop. There are chopping devices available in most appliance and hardware stores.

COARSELY CHOP Chop in pieces approximately 1/2-inch square.

COAT Using a sifter, sprinkle ingredient with flour, cornmeal, etc., until coated. Or roll in flour or shake in a paper bag until coated.

CODDLE Usually used when referring to eggs. When a raw egg is called for in a recipe such as eggnog, Caesar salad, et cetera, put the egg in boiling water for 30 seconds before using it. The reason for coddling the egg is that avedin, a component of raw egg whites, is believed to block the absorption of biotin, one of the water-soluable vitamins. Avedin is extremely sensitive to heat and coddling the egg inactivates the avedin.

COOL Allow to stand at room temperature until no longer warm to the touch.

CORE Remove core from fruits such as pears and apples.

COVER TIGHTLY Seal so that steam cannot escape.

CREAM With a spoon, rub against sides of bowl until creamy. A pastry blender may also be used.

CRUMBLE Crush with your hands or a fork into crumblings.

CRUSH Crush dry herbs with a mortar and pestle before using.

CUBE Cut into cube-shaped pieces approximately 1 inch or specified size.

DEEP FRY Use a deep-fat fryer and add enough oil to cover food to be cooked. If temperature is given in the recipe, a deep-fat frying thermometer will be needed.

DICE Cut into 1/4-inch cubes or smaller.

DISSOLVE Mix dry ingredients with liquid until no longer visible in the solution.

DOT Scatter in small bits over surface of food, actually "sprinkling." Usually refers to butter or margarine.

DREDGE Sprinkle lightly with flour, or coat with flour.

FILLET Remove all bones; usually refers to fish.

FINELY CHOP Chop in pieces approximately 1/4-inch square.

FOLD IN Using a rubber spatula or spoon in a circular motion coming across the bottom, fold the bottom of a mixture over the top. Repeat slowly until mixture is folded in as indicated in the recipe.

FORK TENDER When food can be easily pierced with a fork.

FRY Cook in a small amount of oil in a skillet.

GRATE Rub the surface to be grated on grater for desired-size particles. Finely grated and coarsely grated foods require two different size graters.

GREASE Rub lightly with margarine, corn oil, etc.

GRIND Use a food chopper or grinder.

JULIENNE CUT Cut in strips approximately 1/4 inch by 2 inches.

KNEAD Usually refers to bread dough. After mixing dough according to recipe, place on a floured surface, flatten ball of dough with floured hands and fold it toward you. With the heels of your hands, press down and flatten again. Continue doing this until dough is smooth and satiny, or as recipe directs.

MARINATE Allow mixture to stand in marinade for length of time indicated in recipe.

MASH Potatoes and many other cooked vegetables can be mashed using a potato masher, or brought to the same consistency in an electric blender or mixer.

MINCE Chop as fine as gravel.

PAN BROIL Cook in ungreased or cured hot skillet, pouring off fat as it accumulates.

PARBOIL Boil in water or other liquid until partially cooked. This usually precedes another method of cooking.

PARE Using a knife, remove the outer covering of foods such as apples and peaches.

PEEL Remove outer covering of foods such as oranges, lemons and bananas.

PIT Remove the pit or seed from fruits such as peaches and plums.

POACH Cook for a short time in simmering liquid.

PREHEAT Set oven to desired temperature. Wait until temperature is reached before baking.

PRESS Usually refers to garlic when using a garlic press.

PUREE Put through a fine sieve or food mill, or use an electric blender.

ROAST To bake meat or poultry.

SAUTE Cook in small amount of hot oil in a skillet.

SCALD Heat to just under the boiling point when tiny bubbles begin to form on the sides of the pan. This is also often called "bring to boiling point."

SCORE Using a knife, make shallow cuts or slits on surface of a food.

SCRAPE Scrape to remove outer skin on foods such as carrots and parsnips, or scrape to produce juice in foods such as onions.

SEAR Brown surface rapidly over high heat in a hot skillet.

SEED Completely remove small seeds from such foods as tomatoes, cucumbers and bell peppers.

SHRED Slice thinly in two directions, or use a shredder.

SIFT Put flour, sugar, etc. through a flour sifter or sieve.

SIMMER Cook just below boiling point (about 185°F at sea level).

SINGE Usually refers to poultry. Hold over flame to burn off all feathers or hairs.

SKEWER Hold together with metal or wooden skewers, or spear chunks of meat/vegetables on wooden skewers, as for shish kabob.

SKIN Remove skin of such foods as chicken; sometimes used when referring to onions.

SLICE Using a sharp knife, slice through evenly to specified thickness.

SNIP Cut into small pieces using scissors or kitchen shears.

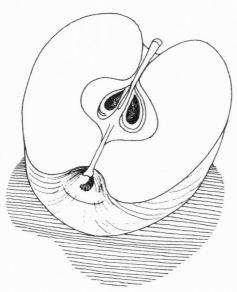

SPRINKLE Just as the word implies, sprinkle, using your fingers as directed in recipe.

STEAM Cook food over boiling water, using either a steamer or a large kettle with a rack placed in the bottom of it to hold the pan or dish of food above the boiling water.

STEEP Allow to stand in hot liquid.

STIFF BUT NOT DRY This term is often used for egg whites and means they should form soft, well-defined peaks but not be beaten to the point where the peaks look as though they will break.

STIFFLY BEATEN Beat until mixture stands in stiff peaks.

STIR Mix with a spoon in a circular motion until all ingredients are well blended.

THICKEN Mix a thickening agent such as arrowroot, cornstarch, flour, etc., with a small amount of liquid to be thickened, then add slowly to the hot liquid, stirring constantly. Cook until slightly thickened or until mixture coats a metal spoon.

THINLY SLICE Using the slicing side of a four-sided grater, slice vegetables such as cucumbers and onions.

TOAST Brown in a toaster, oven or under a broiler. Nuts, seeds or coconut may be toasted in a 350°F oven until desired color is attained. Or, place under broiler and watch carefully, as they burn quickly.

TOSS Mix from both sides in an under-and-over motion toward the center, using two spoons or a fork and spoon; usually refers to salads.

WHIP Beat rapidly with fork, whisk, egg beater or electric mixer to add air and increase volume of mixture.

WHISK Stir, beat or fold using a wire whisk.

Equivalents

BEVERAGES
Ice cubes
2 ice cubes = 1/4 cup
8 ice cubes = 1 cup
Instant coffee
4-ounce jar = 60 cups coffee
Coffee
1 pound (80 tablespoons) = 40 to
50 cups
Tea leaves
1 pound = 300 cups tea

BREADS
Crumbs
Bread crumbs, soft, 1 slice = 3/4 cup
Bread crumbs, dry, crumbled, 2 slices
=1/2 cup
Bread crumbs, dry, ground, 4 slices =
1/2 cup
Graham crackers, 14 squares, fine
crumbs = 1 cup
Soda crackers, 21 squares, fine crumbs
= 1 cup
Cereals and Noodles
Flour, cake, 1 pound = 4-1/2 cups,
sifted
Flour, all-purpose, 1 pound = 4 cups,
sifted
Bulgur, 1/3 cup = 1 cup, cooked
Cornmeal, 1 cup = 4 cups, cooked
Macaroni, 1 pound, 5 cups = 12 cups,
cooked
Noodles, 1 pound, 5-1/2 cups =
10 cups, cooked
Oatmeal, 1 cup = 2 cups, cooked;
1-1/2 cups ground = 1 cup oat flour
Spaghetti, 1 pound = 9 cups, cooked

FATS
Miscellaneous
Bacon, 1 pound, rendered = 1-1/2 cups
Bacon, 1 slice, cooked crisp = 1 table-
spoon, crumbled

Butter, 1 cube (1/4 pound) = 1/2 cup
or 8 tablespoons
Cheese, cream, 3-ounce package =
6 tablespoons
Cream, heavy whipping, 1 cup =
2 cups, whipped
Margarine, 1 cube (1/4 pound) =
1/2 cup or 8 tablespoons
Nuts in the shell
Almonds, 1 pound = 1 cup nutmeats
Brazil nuts, 1 pound = 1-1/2 cups
nutmeats
Peanuts, 1 pound = 2 cups nutmeats
Pecans, 1 pound = 2-1/2 cups nutmeats
Walnuts, 1 pound = 2-1/2 cups
nutmeats
Nuts, shelled
Almonds, 1/2 pound = 2 cups
Almonds, 56, chopped = 1/2 cup
Brazil nuts, 1/2 pound = 1-1/2 cups
Coconut, 1/2 pound, shredded =
2-1/2 cups
Macadamia nuts, 3, finely chopped =
1 tablespoon
Peanuts, 1/2 pound = 1 cup
Peanuts, 50, chopped = 1/2 cup
Pecans, 1/2 pound = 2 cups
Pecans, 42 halves, chopped = 1/2 cup
Walnuts, 1/2 pound = 2 cups
Walnuts, 15 halves, chopped = 1/2 cup

FRUITS (DRIED)
Apricots, 24 halves, 1 cup = 1-1/2
cups, cooked
Dates, 1 pound, 2-1/2 cups = 1-3/4
cups, pitted and chopped; 12 dates,
pitted and chopped = 1/2 cup
Figs, 1 pound, 2-1/2 cups = 4-1/2
cups, cooked
Pears, 1 pound, 3 cups = 5-1/2 cups,
cooked
Prunes, pitted, 1 pound, 2-1/2 cups =
3-3/4 cups, cooked
Raisins, seedless, 1 pound, 2-3/4 cups
= 3-3/4 cups, cooked

FRUITS (FRESH)
Apples, 1 pound, 4 small = 3 cups,
chopped
Apricots, 1 pound, 6 to 8 average =
2 cups, chopped
Bananas, 1 pound, 4 small = 2 cups,
mashed
Berries, 1 pint = 2 cups
Cantaloupe, 2 pounds, 1 average =
3 cups, diced
Cherries, 1 pint = 1 cup, pitted
Cranberries, 1 pound = 4-1/2 cups
Crenshaw melon, 3 pounds,
1 average = 4-1/2 cups, diced
Figs, 1 pound, 4 small = 2 cups,
chopped
Grapefruit, 1 small = 1 cup, sectioned
Grapes, Concord, 1/4 pound, 30 grapes
= 1 cup
Grapes, Thompson seedless, 1/4
pound, 40 grapes = 1 cup
Guavas, 1 pound, 4 medium = 1 cup,
chopped
Honeydew melon, 2 pounds, 1 average
= 3 cups, diced
Kumquats, 1 pound, 8 to 10 average
= 2 cups, sliced
Lemon, 1 medium (3 average =
1 pound) = 3 tablespoons juice;
2 teaspoons grated peel
Limes, 1/2 pound, 5 average = 4 tablespoons juice; 4 to 5 teaspoons
grated peel
Loquats, 1 pound, 5 average = 1-1/2
cups, chopped
Lychees, 1 pound, 6 average = 1/2
cup, chopped
Mangoes, 1 pound, 2 average = 1-1/2
cups, chopped
Nectarines, 1 pound, 3 average =
2 cups, chopped
Orange, 1 small (2 average = 1 pound)
= 6 tablespoons juice; 1 tablespoon
grated peel, 3/4 cup sectioned
Papaya, 1 medium = 1-1/2 cups,
chopped

Peaches, 1 pound, 3 average = 2 cups, chopped

Pears, 1 pound, 3 average = 2 cups, chopped

Persimmons, 1 pound, 3 average = 2 cups, mashed

Pineapple, 3 pounds, 1 medium = 2-1/2 cups, chopped

Plums, 1 pound, 4 average = 2 cups, chopped

Pomegranate, 1/4 pound, 1 average = 3 cups seeds

Prunes, 1 pound, 5 average = 2 cups, chopped

Rhubarb, 1 pound, 4 slender stalks = 2 cups, cooked

Tangerines, 1 pound, 4 average = 2 cups, sectioned

Watermelon, 10 to 12 pounds, 1 average = 20 to 24 cups, cubed

HERBS, SPICES AND SEASONINGS

Garlic powder, 1/8 teaspoon = 1 small clove garlic

Ginger, powdered, 1/2 teaspoon = 1 teaspoon, fresh

Herbs, dried, 1/2 teaspoon = tablespoon, fresh

Horseradish, bottled, 2 tablespoons = 1 tablespoon, fresh

MEATS

Cheese

Cottage cheese, 1/2 pound = 1 cup

Cheese, grated, 1/4 pound = 1 cup

Eggs and Egg Substitutes

Eggs, raw, whole, 6 medium = 1 cup

Eggs, raw, in shell, 10 medium = 1 pound

Egg whites, 1 medium = 1-1/2 tablespoons

Egg whites, 9 medium = 1 cup

Egg yolks, 1 medium = 1 tablespoon

Egg yolks, 16 medium = 1 cup

Egg, hard-cooked, 1 = 1/3 cup, finely chopped

Egg substitute, liquid, 1/4 cup = 1 egg (see label)

Egg substitute, dry, 3 tablespoons = 1 egg (see label)

Seafood and Fish

Crab, fresh or frozen, cooked or canned, 1/2 pound (5-1/2- to 7-1/2-ounce tin) = 1 cup

Escargots, 6 snails = 1-1/2 ounces

Lobster, fresh or frozen, cooked, 1/2 pound = 1 cup

Oysters, raw, 1/2 pound = 1 cup

Scallops, fresh or frozen, shucked, 1/2 pound = 1 cup

Shrimp, cooked, 1 pound = 3 cups

Tuna, drained, canned, 6-1/2 to 7 ounces = 3/4 cup

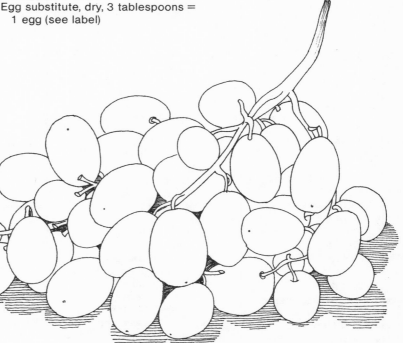

MILK

Dry, whole powdered milk, 1/4 cup +
1 cup water = 1 cup whole milk

Dry, instant non-fat powdered milk,
1/3 cup + 2/3 cup water = 1 cup
non-fat milk

Dry, non-instant non-fat powdered
milk, 3 tablespoons + 1 cup water =
1 cup non-fat milk

Skimmed, canned, 1 cup = 5 cups,
whipped

STOCK BASE AND BOUILLON CUBES

Beef Stock Base, Powdered

1 teaspoon = 1 bouillon cube

4 teaspoons + 1-1/4 cups water =
1 10-1/2-ounce can bouillon,
undiluted

1 teaspoon + 5 ounces water =
5 ounces stock

1 teaspoon + 1 cup water = 1 cup
bouillon

Chicken Stock Base, Powdered

1 teaspoon = 1 bouillon cube

1 teaspoon + 5 ounces water =
5 ounces stock

1 teaspoon + 1 cup water = 1 cup
bouillon

VEGETABLES (DRIED)

Garbanzo beans, 1 pound, 2 cups =
6 cups, cooked

Kidney beans, 1 pound, 1-1/2 cups =
9 cups, cooked

Lima or navy beans, 1 pound, 2-1/2
cups = 6 cups, cooked

Rice, 1 pound, 2-1/2 cups = 8 cups,
cooked

Split peas, 1 pound, 2 cups = 5 cups,
cooked

VEGETABLES (FRESH)

Artichokes, 1/2 pound = 1 average

Asparagus, 1 pound, 18 spears =
2 cups, cut in 1-inch pieces

Avocado, 1 medium = 2 cups, chopped

Beans, green, 1 pound = 3 cups,
chopped and cooked

Beets, 1 pound, medium-size = 2 cups,
cooked and sliced

Bell pepper, 1/2 pound, 1 large = 1 cup
seeded and finely chopped

Broccoli, 1 pound, 2 stalks = 6 cups,
chopped and cooked

Brussels sprouts, 1 pound, 28 average
= 4 cups

Cabbage, 1 pound = 4 cups, shredded;
2-1/2 cups, cooked

Carrots, 1 pound, 8 small = 4 cups,
chopped

Cauliflower, 1-1/2 pounds, 1 average
= 6 cups, chopped and cooked

Celery, 1 stalk = 1/2 cup, finely chopped

Celery root, 1-3/4 pounds, 1 average
= 4 cups raw, grated; 2 cups cooked
and mashed

Corn, 6 ears = 1-1/2 cups, cut

Cucumber, 1 medium = 1-1/2 cups,
sliced

Eggplant, 1 pound, 1 medium = 12
1/4-inch slices; 6 cups, cubed

Lettuce, 1 average head = 6 cups,
bite-size pieces

Lima beans, baby, 1 pound = 2 cups

Mushrooms, fresh, 1/2 pound, 20
medium = 2 cups raw, sliced

Okra, 24 medium = 1/2 pound

Onion, 1 medium = 1 cup, finely
chopped

Parsnips, 1 pound, 6 average = 4
cups, chopped

Peas, in pods, 1 pound = 1 cup, shelled
and cooked

Pimiento, 1 4-ounce jar = 1/2 cup,
chopped

Potatoes, 1 pound, 4 medium = 2-1/2
cups, cooked and diced

Pumpkin, 3 pounds, 1 average piece
= 4 cups, cooked and mashed

Rutabagas, 1-1/2 pounds, 3 small =
2 cups, cooked and mashed

Spinach, 1 pound = 3-1/2 cups, uncooked; 1 cup, cooked

Squash, acorn, 1-1/2 pounds, 1 average
= 2 cups, cooked and mashed

Squash, banana, 3 pounds, 1 average
piece = 4 cups, cooked and mashed

Squash, spaghetti, 1 medium =
4 cups, cooked

Squash, summer, 1 pound, 4 average
= 1 cup, cooked

Squash, zucchini, 1 pound, 2 average
= 1-1/4 cups, cooked and chopped;
3 cups raw, diced

Tomatoes, 1 pound, 3 medium = 1-1/4
cups, cooked and chopped

Turnips, white, 1 pound, 3 small =
2 cups, peeled and grated;
1-1/4 cups cooked and mashed

MISCELLANEOUS

Chocolate, 1 square, 1 ounce = 4
tablespoons, grated

Gelatin, sheet, 4 sheets = 1 envelope

Gelatin, powdered, 1/4-ounce envelope
= 1 scant tablespoon

Yeast, fresh, 1 package = 2 tablespoons

Yeast, dry, 1 envelope (to be reconsti-
tuted in 2 tablespoons water) = 1-3/4
tablespoons

METRIC WEIGHTS

For Dry Measure

Convert known ounces into grams by
multiplying by 28

Convert known pounds into kilograms
by multiplying by .45

Convert known grams into ounces by
multiplying by .035

Convert known kilograms into pounds
by multiplying by 2.2

For Liquid Measure

Convert known ounces into milliliters
by multiplying by 30

Convert known pints into liters by
multiplying by .47

Convert known quarts into liters by
multiplying by .95

Convert known gallons into liters by
multiplying by 3.8

Convert known milliliters into ounces
by multiplying by .034

Bibliography

Biermann, June, and Toohey, Barbara. *The Diabetic's Total Health Book.* Los Angeles: J. P. Tarcher, 1980.

Bowes and Church. *Food Values of Portions Commonly Used,* 13th ed. New York: Harper and Row, 1980.

"Composition of Foods: Raw, Processed, Prepared." *Revised U.S.D.A. Agricultural Handbook,* no. 8, 1975.

"Dietary Goals for the United States." *U.S. Senate Select Committee on Nutrition and Human Needs,* 2nd ed., December 1977.

"Disease Prevention and Health Promotion: Federal Programs and Prospects." *Report of the Departmental Task Force on Prevention.* U.S. Department of Health, Education and Welfare, September 1978.

"Healthy People—The Surgeon General's Report on Health Promotion and Disease Prevention, Background Papers." U.S. Department of Health, Education and Welfare, 1979.

Jones, Jeanne. *The Calculating Cook,* rev. ed. San Francisco: 101 Productions, 1978.

Jones, Jeanne. *Diet for a Happy Heart,* rev. ed. San Francisco: 101 Productions, 1981.

Jones, Jeanne. *Fabulous Fiber Cookbook.* San Francisco: 101 Productions, 1979.

Jones, Jeanne. *Secrets of Salt-Free Cooking.* San Francisco: 101 Productions, 1979.

Jones, Jeanne, and Kientzler, Karma. *Fitness First: A 14-Day Diet and Exercise Program.* San Francisco: 101 Productions, 1980.

"Nutritive Value of American Foods in Common Units." *U.S.D.A. Agricultural Handbook,* no. 456, 1975.

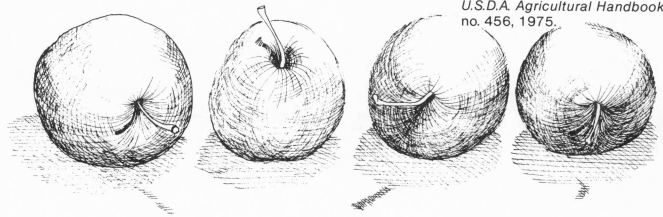

Index

Biographical Notes

Jeanne Jones

Jeanne Jones is recognized as one of the leading writers, lecturers and consultants in the diet field. Her imaginative approach to entertaining, menu planning, food preparation and presentation has gained her an international reputation as a hostess. Her first book, *The Calculating Cook,* was published in 1972, followed by *Diet for a Happy Heart* (1975), *The Fabulous Fiber Cookbook* (1977), *Secrets of Salt-Free Cooking* (1979), *Jeanne Jones' Party Planner and Entertaining Diary* (1979), *The Fabulous Fructose Recipe Book* (1979, co-authored with J. Thomas Cooper, M.D.) and *Fitness First: A 14-Day Diet and Exercise Program* (1980, co-authored with Karma Kientzler).

She serves as a consultant on recipe and menu planning and new product development for a number of health organizations, food manufacturers, health resorts and restaurants. She has lectured all over the world at professional meetings and has appeared as a guest expert on diet and cooking on over 300 radio and television programs throughout the United States and Canada.

Jeanne is an editorial associate of *Diabetes Forecast,* the official magazine of the American Diabetes Association, and a member of the External Advisory Committee to the Diet Modification Program of the National Heart and Blood Vessel Research Demonstration Center in Houston and the Patient Advisory Committee of the Scripps Clinic and Research Foundation, La Jolla, California. She has served on the board of the Southern California Affiliate of the American Diabetes Association and is currently on the board of the San Diego County Heart Association and is a member of its Nutrition Committee. In 1976, she was chairman of a diet panel for the Ninth International Diabetes Federation Congress in New Delhi, India, and spoke again September 1979, as a member of a panel at the Tenth International Diabetes Federation Congress in Dubrovnik, Yugoslavia.

Holly Zapp

The first book to be illustrated by Holly Zapp was Jeanne Jones' first book, *The Calculating Cook,* and subsequently her drawings have appeared in two other publications of 101 Productions: The 1974 *Kitchen Herb Calendar* and a cookbook entitled *Jams and Jellies* (1975). A graduate in fine arts from Syracuse University, Mrs. Zapp has also animated several films for the Sesame Street television series. She and her husband, Ivar, also an artist, divide their time between San Francisco and Costa Rica.

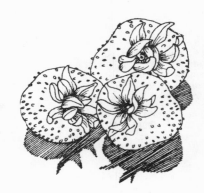